Stop Smoking
for Good

Stop Smoking
for Good

Forget the Patch, the Gum, and the Excuses
with Dr. Prasad's Proven Program for
Permanent Smoking Cessation

Balasa L. Prasad, M.D.

with Catherine Whitney

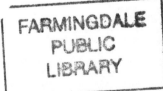
Avery   a member of Penguin Group (USA) Inc.   New York

AVERY

Published by the Penguin Group

Penguin Group (USA) Inc., 375 Hudson Street, New York, New York 10014, U.S.A. • Penguin
Group (Canada), 90 Eglinton Avenue East, Suite 700, Toronto, Ontario M4P 2Y3, Canada
(a division of Pearson Penguin Canada Inc.) • Penguin Books Ltd, 80 Strand, London WC2R 0RL,
England • Penguin Ireland, 25 St Stephen's Green, Dublin 2, Ireland (a division of Penguin Books Ltd) •
Penguin Books (Australia), 250 Camberwell Road, Camberwell, Victoria 3124, Australia (a division
of Pearson Australia Group Pty Ltd) • Penguin Books India Pvt Ltd, 11 Community Centre,
Panchsheel Park, New Delhi–110 017, India • Penguin Group (NZ), Cnr Airborne and Rosedale Roads,
Albany, Auckland 1310, New Zealand (a division of Pearson New Zealand Ltd) • Penguin Books
(South Africa) (Pty) Ltd, 24 Sturdee Avenue, Rosebank, Johannesburg 2196, South Africa

Penguin Books Ltd, Registered Offices: 80 Strand, London WC2R 0RL, England

Library of Congress Cataloging in Publication Data

Prasad, Balasa L.
Stop smoking for good: forget the patch, the gum, and the excuses with Dr. Prasad's proven program
for permanent smoking cessation/Balasa L. Prasad, M.D., with Catherine Whitney.
p. cm.
Includes index.
ISBN 1-58333-234-0
1. Cigarette habit—Psychological aspects. 2. Smoking—Psychological aspects.
3. Smoking cessation programs. I. Whitney, Catherine. II. Title.
HV5740.P73   2005
616.86'506—dc22   2005045314

Printed in the United States of America
3   5   7   9   10   8   6   4

Book design by Meighan Cavanaugh

CONTENTS

This book is dedicated with love and gratitude to:

My parents, especially my mother. She was an extraordinary woman who instilled in me discipline, compassion, and a deep sense of responsibility. She taught me to dream big and work hard to make that dream a reality. She encouraged me to believe in myself, and to do the best I could with my God-given talents.

My wife, Vasantha, who is the love of my life. She has always been a great inspiration for me—highly supportive, constantly encouraging me to work hard and to be proud of everything I do in my profession. She truly is a life partner at home and at work.

My daughter and only child, Bindu, a smart, wonderful young lady who has been my greatest fan and best critic. Bindu has always helped me with remarkable comments and suggestions.

They say that there is a woman behind every successful man, but in my case I feel blessed to have three smart and intuitive women who have helped me come this far in life.

ACKNOWLEDGMENTS

Special thanks to Judge Judy Sheindlin. When I was almost finished with my manuscript, I met Judge Judy, who took a look at it and felt that it had great potential and put me in touch with her publishing agent immediately. I was excited because I have a great deal of respect for Judy. She is one of the most intelligent and astute individuals whom I have had the pleasure of meeting.

Endless thanks to Catherine Whitney, who thoroughly understood my philosophical and scientific approach to dealing with habits. She literally transformed my manuscript into an interesting and enlightening book. She is a wonderful writer, and I feel very lucky to have had the opportunity to work with her.

My thanks to my literary agents, Jane Dystel and Miriam Goderich, who took an early interest in my manuscript and believed in me. They worked tirelessly to see that my book found the right publishing home.

My editors at Avery, Megan Newman and Kristen Jennings, have showed enthusiasm and creativity, and I am proud to have them behind my work. It was Megan who decided to present the material in a series of practical books in order to spread their impact as far as possible. Kristen has shepherded the manuscripts through the process with great sensitivity to my intentions.

Thanks to Dr. Preetham Grandhi, a child and adolescent psychiatrist, who engaged me in a healthy debate about psychiatric views. I am also grateful to the nursing staff at Mount Vernon Hospital in New

York, who served as my spokespeople to my patients and the public. They are and will always be my biggest cheerleaders.

Last but not least, I want to thank my patients of the past twenty-five years who have helped me to strengthen my beliefs and my profound philosophy. They have taught me firsthand that there are no simple answers to life's complex problems. It is very gratifying for me to know that I have been of help to them in dealing with challenges in their day-to-day life, and have played a part in their happiness, health, and success.

INTRODUCTION

A Lesson from My Grandfather

WHEN I WAS A BOY growing up in Bangalore, India, my paternal grandparents who lived nearby came to dinner every week. One of my earliest memories is of my grandfather, seated at the head of the table, smiling, talking, and smoking. I never saw him without a cigarette dangling from his mouth. Smoke curled from his lips as he spoke, and he would extinguish one cigarette only to light another. My grandmother pestered him incessantly to give up his habit, citing the effects of smoking on his health, and she chastised him for setting a bad example for his impressionable grandchildren. She was a remarkably astute woman, as the health effects of smoking were virtually unexamined in the 1950s. My grandmother wisely made the connection between my grandfather's persistent cough and his habit.

Grandfather's smoking was a frequent subject of conversation around our dinner table. When my grandmother's hectoring became too annoying, he would boldly promise to quit the next day. As proof of his intent, he'd present a wager to the grandchildren: "I'll make a bet with you," he'd tell us, with a twinkle in his eye. "If I smoke a cigarette tomorrow, I will pay each of you a quarter. If I don't smoke, you will pay me a quarter." We delighted in this game, as it was quite lucrative for us. The quarters piled up in our pockets, and Grandfather continued to smoke.

One day, when I was ten, the game came to an end. We were seated around the table when Grandfather was overtaken by a severe coughing fit. Grandmother waited until it had subsided, then spoke in a quiet, conciliatory tone that I had never before heard her use. "I hope you live a long life, so you can enjoy the happiness of this family you worked so hard to build," she told Grandfather. "I do not want to be left alone in the world to watch our precious grandchildren grow, and to witness their graduations, marriages, and the births of their children without you by my side. But if you are bent on committing suicide with your cigarettes, there is nothing I can do. I am merely a helpless bystander and well-wisher. I cannot pester you into saving your life."

The table was silent, and I saw the mischievous grin fade from Grandfather's face. Something in Grandmother's quiet plea had struck a chord with him. He stared into her eyes for a long time, then reached over and extinguished his burning cigarette. "My smoking days are over," he announced. We knew he was serious when he refused to take a wager on quitting the habit. "I have no intention of collecting money from my own grandchildren," he said firmly.

My grandfather lived for fourteen more years, and he never touched another cigarette. He did not seem to struggle with the decision or put on weight after he quit. I once asked him if it was hard not to smoke. He shrugged dismissively. "I enjoyed cigarettes for fifty-two years, and it was high time I let go of the pleasure as well as the cigarette," he said.

One thing I will never forget about the night my grandfather stopped smoking was the sudden change in his eyes when he announced his decision. It's no wonder poets proclaim that the eyes are the windows to the soul. The sparkle in my grandfather's eyes revealed a transformation that went beyond fancy words and promises. He was a changed man, just like that.

The incident stayed with me, and I often wondered about the source of that sparkle, which seemed to emanate from his very soul. What had transpired in my grandfather's mind in that instant that allowed him to rise above his usual, lackadaisical manner and summon the strength to turn his back on a lifelong pleasure? When I began my psychiatric practice and started treating patients whose addictions were every bit as tenacious as my grandfather's, I often found myself thinking about that moment, and asking myself what I could learn from it. I entered the field at a time when there was a vast array of treatment options available, including many kinds of chemicals to help people overcome their habits. Yet the most sophisticated state-of-the-art programs and lavish facilities had very high failure rates. Most of my patients had tried them all, and they arrived at my office with a desperation born of repeated failures.

What distinguished these people from my grandfather? He had none of the tools of modern recovery. Indeed, the thought of my grandfather wearing a nicotine patch or attending a support group makes me smile.

But how many people could walk away from a fifty-two-year habit without a second glance back? I know that many people would say that my grandfather must have possessed a remarkable character to make such a dramatic and firm commitment. They would conclude that his strength of purpose was rare. Surely, the average person could not experience such a transformation.

I have discovered exactly the opposite. In the twenty-five years I've worked to help people overcome destructive habits that run the gamut from smoking to drug abuse to obsessive food cravings to sexual excess, I have witnessed similar transformations thousands of times. I am not saying that it is easy for my patients to give up their addictive pleasures. It always requires strength and determination. However, the choice to forgo the comforts and thrills of the addictive behavior becomes natural to them once they taste the greater joys of freedom. Like my grandfather, they are no longer willing to pay such a heavy price to maintain their addictions.

This process, which I will describe in this book, involves a focus on the mind of a smoker, not on the chemical or structural nature of the brain or a person's external behavior. Smoking itself is merely a physical manifestation of a deeper craving triggered by the emotional center of the mind.

Today when I remember my grandfather, I see images from his final fourteen years, after he had snuffed out his last cigarette. He achieved a new stature, a visible happiness. I remember him bursting with pride when I graduated from medical school, beaming with the joy of a life well lived and the satisfaction of watching his progeny take flight. He died with a smile of satisfaction on his face. Without realizing it, my grandfather taught me a vital lesson about human fulfillment. My mission is to pass this lesson on to as many people as I can. Our time on this earth is short. We are but brief flashes of light on eternity's landscape, but we alone among all of God's creatures have a chance to feel the wonder of that light.

Part One

The Smoker's Mind

There Are No Nicotine Addicts

SEVERAL YEARS AGO I conducted a small experiment to test my hypothesis that nicotine addiction is not the primary reason people continue to smoke. I chose twenty hard-core smokers at random and switched their cigarette brands. Even though the new brands contained the same amount of nicotine, all of the smokers experienced mild-to-moderate withdrawal symptoms in the first couple of days. They reported not getting the same satisfaction from these different brands. It took on average six weeks for them to achieve the same level of comfort they'd had with their old brands. The response was even more pronounced when smokers of mentholated cigarettes were switched to nonmentholated brands. These smokers struggled a lot harder than the others. Several found that they could not stay on the nonmentholated brands longer than three or four days.

This experiment confirmed what I had observed among thousands of patients: the pleasure perception experienced by most smokers is not related to the chemical substance nicotine. Here's the million-dollar question: if nicotine is not the true culprit in giving pleasure, then what compels a person to be chained to this habit?

The Pleasure of Smoking

In the first instance, the pleasure derived from smoking comes from the warm, velvety smoke, laced with the resin of the tobacco leaf, which excites the delicate mucous membranes of the air passages. This sensation is the reason why smokers experience maximum pleasure from the first cigarette in the morning, and those cigarettes smoked after do not carry the same punch. During the night, the mucous membranes have time to recover and regain their sensitivity. Even a short smoke-free interval helps to heal the mucous membranes, translating into a heightened pleasure perception.

Smokers are addicted to the titillating effect of the smoke from a cigarette, rather than the stimulating effects of nicotine. The pleasure of the warm smoke caressing the trachea and the bronchi is the enticing factor and the driving force behind their habit. As my experiment demonstrated, most smokers are intensely sensitive to the quality of the smoke they draw into their lungs. A small percentage prefer only mentholated cigarettes because the quality of the smoke from these cigarettes is different from that of the nonmentholated brands. Menthol adds a cool touch to the smoke. The lungs become used to this smoke, and the nonmentholated brands do not give them the same pleasure.

Unlike cocaine, which is a powerful stimulant and a euphoric agent, nicotine is only a mild stimulant with a very weak euphoric effect. A standard dose of nicotine, ranging from 2.5 to 6 milligrams, produces a slight buzz. Many low-tar, low-nicotine cigarettes contain less than 1 milligram of nicotine. A new smoker may feel light-headed or alert, but experience no euphoria. Hence nicotine alone isn't responsible for the powerful draw. At higher doses, far from causing a pleasurable sensation, nicotine can produce dizziness and palpitations, blurred vision, and headaches. At 60 milligrams, which is considered toxic, nicotine triggers irregular heartbeat, leading to low blood pressure, convulsions, and coma. Amounts above 60 milligrams are considered lethal.

Consider this: no one comes into this world with a cigarette dangling from his mouth. Indeed, the first puff of smoke initially shocks the body. It is a most unwelcome intrusion. If you've ever observed a person violently coughing after inhaling his first cigarette, you know what I mean. After a few exposures, the body grudgingly accommodates the intrusion, although it never fully accepts it. If this is so, why can't the smoker easily stop? Most people explain it by saying that nicotine has an addictive hold on them. They want to stop, but they're chemically forced to continue. That explanation fails to solve the major puzzle about the smoking addiction: why the smoker remains tied to the habit for years after the chemical has completely left the body. Many people who quit smoking report that months or even years after stopping, they retain the compulsion to smoke, and a high percentage ultimately return to smoking.

To solve this puzzle we must shift our focus from the nicotine to the smoker. There is no question that over time a deep relationship develops between the smoker and cigarettes—even a sense of trust. Smoking becomes part of users' lifestyle, an extension of their personality. Nicotine is not the culprit; there are deeper forces at work.

Every human being is born with the potential to become an addict because we are all inherently pleasure seekers. If you eliminate the constant fear for survival, which we have effectively done in most modern societies, the pursuit of pleasure becomes dominant. However, most people recognize that they must rein in their pleasure-seeking behaviors and approach them with moderation. This self-regulation becomes second nature for most of us. We do not have to struggle every minute to deny ourselves pleasure. If there is a quart of ice cream in the freezer, we can eat a serving without feeling an overwhelming urge to finish off the whole thing. Likewise, most people are not driven to take mind-altering drugs or to drink excessively. If they experiment with these behaviors, they frequently find that the discomfort far outweighs any pleasure.

Furthermore, since humans are social animals, most of us are constrained by cultural standards. For example, Indian society considers it taboo for women to smoke cigarettes; consequently, there are few women smokers. Alcohol has also traditionally been stigmatized. When I was growing up, the upper and middle classes viewed alcohol with contempt. Alcohol consumption was associated almost entirely with the poor labor class, which would get buzzed on cheap liquor after a hard day's work. Fearful of being identified with the crass habits of the lower classes, the rest of society stayed away from alcohol. It would have been shameful to be caught holding a glass of beer. In the last twenty years, these attitudes have softened considerably, and as a result, the problems of alcoholism are making their way into upper- and middle-class Indian households. We cannot ignore the powerful influence the culture exerts in making addictive behaviors acceptable.

Compared to other destructive habits, the social consequences of smoking have not always been immediately apparent. The cost, job loss, family breakups, and financial disaster do not threaten from the moment a person takes his first puff. Even health damages do not appear for many years. Chronic inflammatory lung disease, organ destruction, and the carcinogenic effects on the body may not occur for decades, giving smokers a false sense of wellness. In recent years, as we have developed a better understanding of the public health risk of smoking, social consequences and legal restrictions have gained prominence. The resulting inconvenience of smoking in public places, heavy taxation and monetary expense, and treatment of smokers as social pariahs have done the most to dislodge smokers from their habits—not the patch, drugs, or hypnosis.

The Problem of Drug Therapy and Nicotine Replacement Treatments

The belief that withdrawal symptoms can be minimized or eliminated through the use of powerful drugs, skin patches, and other nicotine replacements is pure folly. These methods may provide a brief relief for some smokers. But many smokers are surprised that the withdrawal symptoms and the strong urge to smoke reappear in one to two weeks. While a chemical tune-up of the brain in a controlled environment may yield temporary results, it will ultimately fail unless the basic addictive mentality is addressed. Time and time again I have treated smokers who spent months and even years smoke-free after treatment. But in every case, the hold of smoking in the mind—the memory of its comfort-giving power—reappeared in stressful situations.

Proponents of drug therapy (such as antidepressants and tranquilizers) and nicotine replacement disregard the depth of dependence and the strong influence of the habit over the daily activities of the smoker. By definition, an addictive habit has an undeniable, overwhelming dominance over an individual. By design, its removal leaves an in-depth emptiness or void, and a strong sense of deprivation in one's mind, which is responsible for most of the withdrawal symptoms. An attempt to offset the psychological withdrawal symptoms with chemical replacements sends the smoker into a tailspin. There is only one way to escape the wrath of deprivation: a smoker must forgo the pleasure, comfort, thrill, and advantages of smoking, and invoke a change in the mind about the value of smoking.

Even if nicotine were the main culprit of this habit (which it is not), Nicorette gum and the patch would be the worst inventions and biggest flops of our era. Think about it. If, as everyone assumes, a smoker is hooked on nicotine, what is the rationale for providing the exact same chemical substance in a different form? Experts contend that by changing the form of administration and gradually decreasing the dosage from 21 milligrams to 14 milligrams to 7 milligrams, as in the case of the patch, the smoker can be comfortably weaned from the habit. However, these methods have failed miserably.

Often smokers using a gradual tapering technique feel as if they are suddenly quitting cold turkey when they reach the last leg of their struggle. Many smokers I have treated who tried to get off cigarettes without the use of aids were easily able to decrease their consumption by 60 percent, but it got tougher toward the end when they had to give up the last few cigarettes. This effect is contrary to the theory behind nicotine replacement methods: if a smoker depended on a certain blood nicotine level for satisfaction, then it should be tougher at the beginning, when the number of cigarettes was drastically cut down from 100 to 40 percent, than at the end. However, my patients tell me that even when they stayed on a reduced number of cigarettes for six to eight weeks, they still experienced the strongest withdrawal symptoms when they came down from the last puff to no puff. For this reason, many smokers like to stay on five to six cigarettes a day. Unfortunately, it is not possible to maintain this level on a permanent basis. It takes continuous vigilance to sustain a change from two packs a day to five cigarettes a day, and this cannot be maintained indefinitely. Once their attention is distracted from the habit, consumers usually pick up the pace.

My patients who have tried the patch have told me many similar stories. In the beginning, the patch helped to decrease the urges to a comfortable level, but users found the urges usually resurfaced in a short period in spite of their using the patch. One patient went back from 14 milligrams to the original dose of 21 milligrams to curb the desire. To his amazement, the 21-milligram patch failed to control the urges the second time. Another patient gave up smoking while using the patch, but a year after the last puff he went back to his old habit. He opted to use the patch again. The second time, however, the patch failed to control his urges and withdrawal symptoms. He was disgusted because he could not even reduce the consumption, proving once again that the nicotine theory is flawed.

Not only do nicotine replacement systems fail to help smokers quit, they may actually play a role in further embedding the habit in the mind of a smoker. Most people who used the nicotine patch have told me it made it easier to stop smoking for one week for sure, and in some cases two or three weeks. After that, they began to miss smoking, and would eventually return. But the urge isn't caused by the call of nicotine. It's the call of the emotions and instinct.

It appears to me that after decades of intense research on the subject of the smoking habit, the role of nicotine and the extent of its influence on a smoker remain unclear. After observing thousands of smokers in my office for more than twenty years, I must dispute the mainstream concept on the subject of nicotine. In my opinion, it has sent the wrong signals to the smokers as well as to the industry involved in antismoking devices. I consider nicotine to be the scapegoat of this century. Although I can understand the temptation to find a straightforward, simplified answer to the unreasonable hardships smokers endure on their journey to freedom from this habit, I believe we have steered wildly off course.

Discovering the Drive to Smoke

Recently, neuroscientists at Columbia Presbyterian Medical Center in New York City were able to demonstrate at a molecular level nicotine's ability to increase the synaptic transmission by intensifying the flow of glutamate, one of the most powerful neurotransmitters in the brain. These researchers are hoping to find a chemical agent that can neutralize the effects of nicotine at the cellular level and help a smoker kick the habit. Unfortunately, even if they are able to find such a safe, nicotine-specific blocking agent, it will be of little value to the established smoker. Why? Because there is no chemical agent that can selectively erase the memories of the pleasure, comfort, and ambience of smoking, which are deeply embedded in the emotional memory bank. Nor can any chemical agent undo the psychological drives that initiate the smoking action. These drives are embedded in emotional memories that will not yield to chemical intervention. They persist even in the absence of pleasure.

Shirley,* a thirty-seven-year-old business executive and mother of a five-year-old, strode into my office, exuding confidence. As she told me about herself, I was impressed. Here was an organized, driven, bright individual. She was extremely successful in her career and was married to a prominent television producer. They had a wonderful child, a lovely home, and a happy life. Shirley told me that she smoked two to three cigarettes a day and wanted to quit altogether.

This was new for me. I had never had anyone walk into my office for help in giving up a couple of cigarettes a day. I asked Shirley if she was sure she wanted to pay a professional for this. "Frankly, you seem to have everything pretty well together," I said.

She smiled wanly. "Dr. Prasad, this is my struggle. All of my adult life I have smoked a few cigarettes a day. I've never gone over a half a pack. The only time I stopped was when I was pregnant with my son."

"Was that difficult for you?" I asked.

She shook her head. "No, not at all. I didn't have withdrawal symptoms or even think about it. But as soon as I finished breast-feeding, I resumed smoking a few cigarettes a day. I smoke one cigarette with my morning coffee, one after dinner, and one before bed. Sometimes I have a cigarette in the afternoon."

I studied Shirley carefully. "You seem healthy and fit," I said, and she nodded. "So what is driving your desire to quit?"

"I want to do it for my child," she said. "I don't smoke

*Names have been changed to protect the privacy of my patients.

around him, but I never want him to see me smoke even a single cigarette. I've been trying to stop for two years. My husband just doesn't understand why I can't. Last year I tried the patch, but I became a maniac when I gave up those last three cigarettes—very bitter and angry. After a week I went back. I get so pissed off when I stop. You are my last hope."

I had rarely seen a person who struggled so violently with her smoking habit, yet Shirley only smoked three cigarettes a day. What was wrong with this picture? Something was, and I knew it wasn't nicotine. I asked Shirley to tell me about her habit. She said that she started smoking when she was twenty-four and in graduate school—very late to pick up the habit. She had never smoked more than a few cigarettes a day.

I asked about her husband, and Shirley said she met him when she was twenty-nine. A friend set them up on a blind date. "I was sitting in the restaurant, smoking a cigarette, and he walked in with this dazzling smile on his face," she recalled. "We dated for eight months, and he never said a word about my occasional cigarette. Then we were married, and the day we returned from our honeymoon he turned to me and said in a very stern and imperious way, 'Now that we're married, I insist that you stop smoking.' I was completely taken aback by his tone and his statement. I shouted at him, 'How dare you! You never said a word about my smoking before.' He just shrugged and said, 'We weren't married before.' I was so outraged. It wasn't the issue of stopping smoking. It was the tone he used—like I was a bad child. I refused to let him control me."

I noticed that Shirley was shaking with anger at the mere recollection of that incident. I smiled at her and said, "Now I understand your problem. Every time you go below three cigarettes, you are compelled to rebel against being controlled. You hear your husband's voice—that tone he used."

Shirley had calmed down, and now she was looking at me with a strange little smile playing on her lips. "How stupid of me," she said quietly. "Of course, that's it." She sighed. "I love my husband very much, and that was probably the only time he ever used that tone with me. I'm not going to fall for this silly trap anymore."

I nodded. "You don't need my treatment. You just needed that clarification."

Shirley brightened. "You know, Doctor, I believe you're right." She rose, gave my hand a hearty shake, and walked out of the office.

Several months later, Shirley called me. "I wanted to let you know that I haven't touched a cigarette since I saw you," she said proudly. "My marriage is better, too. You see, even though we were happily married, there was always something nagging at me in the back of my mind—a discomfort that I couldn't pinpoint and couldn't shake. I now know it was that incident, which was burned into all of my senses. Now that I've let it go, I feel remarkably free."

Shirley was a prime example of an individual who is caught up in the drive to smoke. Yet her addiction had little if anything to do with the chemical substance nicotine.

In the beginning of my career, I, too, was under the impression that nicotine played a pivotal role in a smoker's life. But time and time again, my patients have proved me wrong. Nicotine is clearly a red herring in this case. The performance of antismoking devices based on the nicotine principle, such as Nicorette gum, gradual filters, and the famous nicotine patch, has consistently failed to measure up to our expectations. Group therapy like SmokEnders or acupuncture, where no chemical adjuncts are advocated, has fared a lot better and has been approved by many smokers as an effective deterrent over that of nicotine substitutes. A psycho-emotional approach to treat an addictive habit has always proved far superior and effective over the physical devices targeting the chemical substance involved in that specific addiction.

There is more to the smoking habit than meets the eye. It is not merely the result of a chemical reaction and a neural response in the brain. It is initiated by the human drive to pursue pleasure and comfort. This drive leads to the initial exposure. But why does one person take a puff and turn away, while another begins the journey to full-fledged addiction? What's really going on here?

2

A Problem of the Mind, Not the Brain

"DR. PRASAD, why do I continue to smoke when I know it's self-destructive? I'm infuriated that this stupid little stick of organic matter has so much power over me."

I observed my patient across the desk. Susan was a vibrant, fit woman in her mid-fifties, a popular television star whose daytime show was number one in the ratings. Her reputation for savvy and smarts was well earned. Everything about her exuded confidence and control, but she couldn't succeed at this one thing so crucial to her health and well-being. Before coming to me, Susan had tried every method available to stop smoking, including the patch, acupuncture, hypnosis, Zyban, nicotine gum, and inhalers.

Her experience was always the same. She'd quit for a few days or even a few weeks, but instead of having less desire for cigarettes, she only craved them more. When the pressure got too great, she'd return to smoking. A producer on Susan's show told her about me, and she made an appointment.

Two weeks after she walked into my office, Susan was a non-smoker. Today, nearly a year later, she reports having no desire for a cigarette, even on her most stressful days. She has become a *comfortable* nonsmoker. How did Susan succeed? She came to see that it was within the power of her mind to neutralize the control of cigarettes.

The addiction to smoking is a problem of the mind, not of the brain. As any person enslaved by a bad habit will tell you, it is not enough to know intellectually that something is bad for you and should be stopped. Most of my patients are completely baffled by their inability to respond to the most persuasive arguments about the harm their behavior is causing to their health, relationships, careers, and well-being. The reason for this disconnection lies in the complex nature of the mind, which involves the dynamic interplay of three divisions—intellect, emotions, and instinct.

The Intellectual, Emotional, and Instinctual Divisions of the Mind

The Intellectual Division of the mind receives information, then presents it to the Emotional Division for acceptance. The Emotional Division is the real policy maker, the one that calls the shots. When an individual can't break a habit, it is because the Intellectual Division has failed to make its case for giving up the habit to the Emotional Division, which says, "Sorry, I'm not convinced. This behavior feels good to me." Without the support of the Emotional Division, both the Intellect—which executes proper actions to safeguard the individual—and the

Instincts—which control habitual behavior—are incapable of making short- or long-term corrections. The only argument the Emotional Division would accept at this point would be a radical one, such as, "The next puff you take will kill you." This is not realistic and therefore cannot be used as a convincing argument by the Intellect.

The human mind is a most effective, complex, and mysterious entity. It is capable of devising swift, savvy, and ingenious maneuvers to help us survive a harsh and ever-changing world. The mind, whose job it is to protect the interests of the individual, attempts to manipulate environmental forces to its advantage. When it fails to do so, it has no choice but to adapt grudgingly to the environmental requirements in order to survive. Unfortunately, when the environment and the mind do not see eye to eye, the mind suffers, and the individual pays a heavy toll in health, happiness, and even survival. Obviously, the mind has an extremely difficult assignment, with little room for error. Let's examine the interplay among the three divisions to better grasp these complex dynamics.

THE INTELLECTUAL DIVISION

The Intellectual Division harbors the pragmatic component of the mind, which we know as human intelligence. The individual characters of this intelligence are reasoning, judgment, logic, discretion, calculation, imagination, analysis, and anticipation. By virtue of these segments, the Intellectual Division is also known as the rational division of the human mind. It is the most complex, sophisticated, and highly evolved section of the mind. Each and every component of the Intellectual Division exhibits a unique natural gift of its own, which comes in handy in fulfilling the Intellect's responsibility. This responsibility is to absorb and analyze the barrage of information it receives from the environment and to program an appropriate response. It appears that nature has picked each and every one of these components for their distinct talent, and purposefully grouped them together under one banner. This ingenious assortment of incredible characters has boosted the Intellectual Division into the front lines of our struggle for survival.

Utilizing the services of our five senses—sight, smell, hearing, taste, and touch—the Intellectual Division receives a steady stream of divergent messages and information from the environment. The individual components of the Intellectual Division analyze millions of bits of information and prepare an appropriate response. If the input from the environment is processed in the Intellectual Division without any interference or influence from the Emotional Division, the outcome of its analysis would be uniform and universal for everyone. Thus, despite there being a diversified ethnic as well as geographic background, one would expect a stereotyped response to the environment from every human being of similar intellectual caliber. But in reality this is not the case. No two human beings are alike. They do not think the same way or have the same interests. Different human beings see the same set of facts from individual perspectives. This diversity is caused primarily by the influence of the Emotional Division.

The Emotional Division

The Emotional Division, which I consider to be the most powerful, conscious counterpart of the Intellectual Division, accommodates two sets of emotions—primitive and advanced.

Primitive emotions are anger, rage, pain, pleasure, comfort, thrill, fear, fright, and selfishness. These primitive emotions are shared by almost all larger (macroscopic) terrestrial organisms. Advanced emotions are love, caring, affection, passion, compassion, concern, grief, deceit, jealousy, hate, greed, pride, and prejudice. The advanced emotions are shared by animal species of a higher intellectual order. The type and the number of advanced emotions are determined by the level of intelligence of the animal species. Human beings are the sole possessors of all levels of emotions, but the primitive emotions often remain the most potent. Love, affection, compassion, and concern are very refined and usually take a backseat to all others. They tend to lose out in an argument to more powerful, primitive emotions and to their close allies—jealousy, greed, hate, and vengeance. This fact is most evident in the human propensity to wage war.

All human beings are born with the same capacity for expressing emotions, but there is an individual variation in the intensity of the influence that each emotion has on the overall function of the mind. For example, in some people rage and anger may have a stronger influence than compassion and tolerance. Likewise, in others, greed, jealousy, and selfishness may mute the influence of other advanced emotions. Therefore, the Emotional Division is the major deciding factor for the individual differences among human beings. This division is also responsible for the overall disposition, attitude, and outlook of a person. In fact, it is the Emotional Division that generates the necessary drive for all advanced life-forms (animals and humans) to initiate an action. Without emotions, human beings would remain passive reactionaries. With emotions, we are aggressive activists.

The Emotional Division of the human mind shapes our

character and our response to the environment. Just imagine if human beings did not have emotions. We would be reduced to nature-created robots—expressionless, mechanical zombies programmed to survive. To illustrate, suppose a person crashes his car into a group of people, causing many injuries and deaths. Obviously the car, being a mechanical contraption, cannot show any emotion. It is under the control of the driver and does what it is directed to do. The driver, being in possession of an emotional division, might exhibit various responses to having caused an accident, including grief, sorrow, fear, remorse, and self-loathing, among others. The driver may fear for his safety and feel that the dire consequences—physical, legal, financial—are overwhelming. The Emotional Division sets the tone and directs the Intellectual Division to come up with a plan of action. The Intellectual Division may then determine that running from the accident scene is the appropriate response. Fear, an emotion, sets the tone, but the actual flight response is concocted and implemented in the Intellectual Division. In an alternative scenario, the emotions of grief and compassion may lead the Intellectual Division to choose a different action—helping the victims and calling for an ambulance. It is the Emotional Division, not the Intellectual Division, that most sets us apart from lower animals.

THE INSTINCTUAL DIVISION

The Instinctual Division is the unconscious counterpart of the Intellectual and Emotional divisions. This division plays a crucial role in our struggle for survival as it holds the directives from nature. Nature expresses its intent through the Instinctual Divisions via three basic directives: (1) protection of self, (2) preservation of the surrounding environment to support the self, and

THE RAW POWER OF EMOTIONS

In my twenty years of practice, I have repeatedly been amazed by the power of the mind over the course of a habit. One of the most dramatic cases I have seen was that of Marian, a fifty-one-year-old woman desperate to stop smoking. Marian had exhausted every available method to quit, and her case was urgent. She suffered from Raynaud's disease, which is poor circulation in the extremities, and smoking made the condition worse. Her doctor had warned that she could lose parts of her hands and feet.

As Marian and I spoke, I came to see that she was an emotionally fragile woman, very sensitive and sentimental. She seemed to crave comfort, and her story explained her fragility. Marian did not start smoking as a young girl. She disliked cigarettes when she was a teenager. In her mid-twenties she married a career soldier in the U.S. Army. A few months after the wedding, Marian's husband was commissioned to fight in Vietnam. Marian was very upset and fearful of losing her husband in the war. By the time he left, she was two months pregnant. At least she had the consolation of carrying her husband's child.

Unfortunately, in her third month her doctor discovered that Marian had an ectopic pregnancy, and it had to be terminated immediately. She was devastated by the loss of her pregnancy and the possibility that she may have to have a hysterectomy. She became depressed and withdrawn. She began to suffer from severe abdominal pains and diarrhea. The usual treatments using antispasmodics, antidiarrheals, and antidepressants failed to help. A psychiatrist who was treating her suggested she should

(continued)

take up smoking as a therapeutic measure. Needless to say, it was a pretty destructive suggestion, and one cannot imagine a psychiatrist making it today, but cigarettes briefly did the trick, and all of Marian's symptoms disappeared within a few days.

Thirty years later, when her doctors told her she must stop smoking to protect her health, Marian was terrified. Poor woman! She was caught between a rock and a hard place. Marian was one of my toughest patients. She needed a lot of coaxing and comforting before she mustered the courage to face the challenge. She was convinced that severe abdominal pains and diarrhea would result if she gave up cigarettes. In actuality, there was no connection between cigarettes and Marian's symptoms, but because she believed that there was, this was enough to keep her smoking. The power of the emotional connection triggered an instinctual reaction.

On rare occasions I use a placebo in the form of tablets to supplement my treatments. This was one such occasion. I prescribed the tablets, explaining to Marian that they would keep her gastrointestinal system from flaring up when she stopped smoking. In spite of my ingenuity, Marian struggled hard to break her bondage to cigarettes. Finally, she succeeded in giving up the habit without suffering abdominal problems. After she quit, I admitted to Marian that I had used a placebo. By then my small deception didn't bother her. She was a confident non-smoker.

(3) propagation of the self. These fundamental directives from nature are incorporated in our mind as basic instincts—thus, the name Instinctual Division. However, in the case of humans, nature has expanded this division to accommodate countless use-

ful acquired or learned habits. Here's the catch: only when the intellect and the emotions are in harmony can an individual recognize his talents and be able to polish them as tools of survival. Therefore, a pragmatic outlook and a healthy attitude are essential in the struggle for survival.

For lower animals, whose learning capacity is limited by meager intellect and a narrow range of emotions, learned behavior pales when compared to unlearned, primary instinctual behavior. Humans are the opposite. By virtue of a wide array of advanced emotions, sassy primitive emotions, and a powerful and versatile intellect, learned behavior not only overshadows but also modifies unlearned primary behavior. With humans, the interpretation of nature's directives and the choice of acquired habits are largely up to the individual.

The Pleasure Principle

The smoking addiction is fundamentally a pleasure-seeking activity, which seizes control of the Emotional Division. Seeking pleasure in the form of comfort, thrill, elation, euphoria, and orgasm has always had a strong pull on the human emotions. Once the pleasure or thrill from an addictive habit is registered in the emotional memory bank, it is very difficult to erase the experience. Addiction weakens the discretionary modality of the Intellectual Division, and the danger signals become less evident as the pleasure pull increases.

Human beings are unique in nature in their drive for pleasure. Lower species are content to follow nature's dictates to ensure survival and the propagation of the species. Because of their primitive emotions and limited intelligence, this species' interpretation of these tasks is simple, and mostly follows nature's cues. For example, animals engage in sexual activity for the ritualistic compliance of propagation. However, the same task is not handled in such a simple fashion by humans.

We humans have developed an additional feature because of our advanced emotions and powerful intelligence. We are driven to utilize every opportunity to make our lives not only secure but also as pleasant, attractive, and easy as possible. For example, humans generally experience sex as a pleasurable activity more than a tool for propagation. (Even those who claim to have sex strictly for propagation purposes expect it to be pleasurable.) Furthermore, sex is sometimes exploited for personal, material, and monetary gains. Thus, advanced, dominant emotions, such as lust for unlimited power, pleasure, immediate gratification, and greed translate the simple mandate of nature in different ways. These emotions set the internal motivation for sexual activity and pass on the need to the intellect, which complies with appropriate action—e.g., demanding lots of sex, having affairs, forcing sex, and so on. These drives are initiated in the Emotional Division.

The Irrational Nature of Emotional Decision Making

For all practical purposes there is an imaginary, active, selective, and psychogenic barrier, like the Great Wall of China, separating the Intellectual Division from the Emotional Division and the Instinctual Division. This barrier acts as a screening agent for the Emotional Division. Like any effective screener, it fully understands the Emotional Division's needs, requirements, and directives. It screens all incoming messages from the Intellectual Division and lets in only those that appeal to the emotions.

This screening agent is nonexistent at birth and appears sometime during early childhood. In the beginning stages, it is a nonselective weak barrier. As a child grows, the barrier becomes stronger and more selective. By the time the youngster reaches early or midteens, it develops into a full-fledged selective barrier. A fully matured and operational screening agent is anything but a simple, passive barrier. Its structural integrity is guarded by the Intellectual Division, and its functional integrity is controlled by the Emotional Division. The Emotional Division dictates terms to the agent that fulfill its own needs. This arrangement leaves very little room for the Intellectual Division to force its messages through to either the Emotional Division or the Instinctual Division.

When the Emotional Division is in a state of distress or turmoil, it can block messages coming from the Intellectual Division. Rational thought is inhibited by the powerful emotional drives. No wonder when you lose your cool or composure, you cannot think or act straight. Only the Intellectual Division is capable of understanding the world we live in and assessing the situations we encounter. However, because it has only conditional access to the rest of the mind, it is forced to compute its response based on the input from the Emotional Division, which can be irrational.

This interplay has great relevance to productive habits, whether they be playing golf or performing surgery, as well as counterproductive habits, such as smoking. When the Intellectual

Division concludes that continuing to smoke presents a threat to an individual's survival, it takes a Herculean effort to convince the Emotional Division to concur.

Many people who come to my office are disgusted and disenchanted by their inability to stop smoking. In fact, they resent having started and having gotten stuck with this destructive habit in the first place. I don't even have to explain the perils of smoking. My patients are already well aware of them. But their intellects are blocked from receiving these healthy messages by the intransigent Emotional Division, which compels them to continue smoking regardless of the consequences.

My patient Ruth was a sixty-two-year-old woman who had been trying to quit smoking for five years. Before coming to me, she had tried hypnosis, Zyban, the patch, Nicorette gum, and even acupuncture.

"I must have a death wish to smoke two packs a day," she said despairingly, referring to her ever-worsening emphysema. At night she had to have a nebulizer, medication, and an oxygen tank in her room. Nonetheless, she had trouble sleeping and had to prop herself up with three pillows in order to breathe more easily. Four months earlier, an acute bout of bronchitis had landed Ruth in the hospital. She stayed there a week and was determined not to smoke again. One week after returning home, she started smoking a cigarette or two a day, and now she was back to two packs a day.

Ruth was attractive and slender, and only her slight wheeze revealed the depths of her problem. She told me she had worked as an office manager for the same company for almost twenty years, and she enjoyed her work. She had been married for thirty-six years and had been separated from her husband for the past three years. She had two adult children—a daughter, thirty-four, and a son, twenty-four—and they were both doing well. She had good relationships with them and was especially close to her daughter, who had recently given birth to her first grandchild.

Ruth had finally left her husband because he had been unfaithful to her for many years. She had tolerated his affairs while her children were young, but once her son had left home, she threw her husband out.

Ruth had also confided that she was a recovering alcoholic who had not touched a drop of alcohol for thirty years. She'd stopped drinking with the help of AA, and even now she attended AA meetings twice a week. She said she had a lot of friends at AA, and going to the meetings was her primary social activity.

"I wonder, Dr. Prasad, why I was able to stop drinking without much difficulty, but I can't stop smoking," Ruth said.

It did not take me too long to figure out why Ruth had consistently failed in her efforts to quit smoking. I observed that though she was a sensitive individual, she was also stubborn and proud, and I sensed a lot of pent-up anger. When I shared my observations, Ruth agreed that this was a fair characterization. She admitted to feeling angry, hurt, and disenchanted.

"Let's get to the bottom of this," I suggested. Ruth went on with her story.

She was the second of four children, born two years after her older sister. When she was ten, her mother gave birth to a son, and a second son was born two years later. Ruth's father was a blue-collar worker who had not finished high school. Her mother was a traditional homemaker.

In their household, Ruth's father was the real captain of the ship. Everyone followed his orders faithfully. When she was still the youngest child, before her brothers were born, Ruth was her father's pet. She was treated specially at home and would often accompany her father in the evenings when he met his friends in a pub to drink beer and smoke cigarettes. Ruth enjoyed being the favored child—as any child would!—and she became very close to her father. This status lasted until the arrival of her brother when she turned ten.

Before her brother's second birthday he had replaced Ruth as her father's favorite child. She was devastated by what she perceived to be her father's betrayal. How could he just push her aside this way? How could he discard her in favor of a boy? She had trusted him.

Ruth just didn't care anymore. She did poorly at school and had few friends. She often skipped classes and would go off with friends to drink beer and smoke cigarettes. She never finished high school, and by age twenty she was a full-blown alcoholic and cigarette smoker. "Drinking calmed me down and helped me forget the pain," she said. "Cigarettes helped me cope with my life." However, it was clear that Ruth wasn't coping too well. For several years she spent most evenings getting drunk at a bar, often taking strangers home and sleeping with them. She knew that what she was doing was morally wrong and that she'd eventually get hurt if she kept it up. But she didn't care and couldn't control her behavior.

She met and married her husband when she was twenty-one, and she continued to drink excessively, but now she did it at home instead of in bars. Her daughter was born a year later.

When her daughter was two years old, Ruth had a rude awakening. One afternoon, after she'd had a few beers, she took the youngster out in the car and had a small accident. Fortunately, her daughter was not seriously hurt, but the ugly bruise on her head and the close call stunned Ruth. She knew she would never forgive herself if she hurt her daughter. Right then and there she decided to stop drinking, and she joined AA. There was not such a rude awakening with her smoking, however, and Ruth continued to smoke. Even at age sixty-two, her repressed anger at her father was driving her to smoke. She was still spiting him after all those years.

When I gently explained the dynamics of her addiction, for the first time Ruth had a good cry. She could see the truth in my words. "I loved my father, then hated him and felt guilty for hating him," she said. "I couldn't get over it, and now he's gone and nothing can change."

I tried to put things into perspective for Ruth. "Your father was limited in many ways," I told her. "He probably never realized how much he hurt you. Your conflict is deep because once you love someone, those feelings never disappear. You have organized your life around the terrible pull of love and resentment. It is time to put this behind you."

Faced with the truth, Ruth finally was able to lay to rest her inner battle with her father and, with it, the cigarettes that had been fueled by her anger.

3

Creatures of Habit

HAVE YOU EVER LEFT your house wondering whether you had locked the front door or turned on the alarm? Whenever my wife and I go out, she always asks me, "Did you close the garage door?" when we're three miles away from the house. We often end up going back to the house, only to find that the doors are locked, the burglar alarm is on, and the lights are off. For the past twenty-five years, my wife and I have gone through this ritual many times. Likewise, every day my wife hands me a stack of letters to mail, expecting that I will drop them in the mailbox by the main entrance of the hospital where I work. And every evening, she asks me whether I have mailed the letters, and without hesitation I answer, "Of course, honey." But for your information, many times I distinctly do not remember whether or not I dropped the mail into the mailbox. So far we've never heard any complaints from our bill collectors, so I must have mailed the letters!

If you're like me, you spend a lot of time looking for those darned car or house keys. A few minutes ago they were in your hand, and seconds later they disappeared into thin air. My car keys especially love to test my patience by playing hide-and-seek with me. When I'm in a hurry, I can never find my keys. Naturally, the more annoyed I become, the longer it takes to find them. In the process, I find every other key that I have been hunting for in the past, except the one that I need at that moment. To avoid this unnecessary headache, I placed a keypad in our kitchen where the door to our garage is located. At first, it took me some time to adjust to this new habit of hanging keys on it, but before long I hung them up without even thinking about it.

Why is it that we do so many routine things but have no distinct, assured recollection of these activities later on? How come the actions that we have just performed are not registered in our minds? The answer is very simple. By design, we are not supposed to remember these routine activities at a conscious level because we are creatures of habit. Many of us are familiar with this expression, but I wonder how many people really understand what it means to be a creature of habit.

What exactly is a habit? The dictionary refers to a habit as a "way of acting that has become fixed through repetition. Habit implies doing something unconsciously and quite often involuntarily or without forethought as a result of much repetition." This process is embedded in our Instinctual Division.

The Formation of a Habit

Why do habits play such a crucial role in our lives? We live in a world that does not automatically guarantee a comfortable, secure, peaceful, and happy lifestyle for all. Life is an uphill struggle. But nature has graciously bestowed upon us the necessary ammunition in our quest to adapt to the ever-changing world and in meeting the demands placed on us by our immediate environment. Habits are one such gift to help us meet the omnipresent challenges. In a way, habits are like a sixth sense. They play a decisive and complex role in shaping our overall behavior patterns. They become an integral part of our lifestyle and blend with our very identities.

Let's pretend for a moment that we lived in a world without habits. Although we would have the capacity to learn the mechanics of an activity, we would not be able to retain this knowledge. Learning the same tasks again and again is monotonous, time-consuming, and self-defeating. For instance, we would be forever riding bicycles with training wheels and never learn the art of balancing a bicycle. And someone daring enough to ski on a dangerous slope might end up licking his wounds in the hospital. And golf balls would be flying in every direction, except onto the fairways and putting greens. It wouldn't be much fun to watch sports played by eternal amateurs, and we wouldn't have many ski resorts, golf and tennis clubs, or auto races. Without the advantage of habit formation, we would be severely handicapped and restricted to performing very few tasks. Without habits we probably would not have survived the Stone Age.

Habits run the spectrum from best to worst. Interestingly enough, only human beings have to sort out good from bad habits and take extra effort to keep bad ones out of reach. Unlike animals, who rely on nature to select the right habits for them, humans have to pick each habit out of many and learn its mechanics to adopt it. Instead of issuing a wide, predetermined array of primary habits, nature granted us a powerful mind with unlimited imagination and the freedom to select the habits of our choice, so that we could be the masters of our own destiny. Unfortunately, such a privilege does not come free. We are expected to display a great deal of diligence, discipline, responsibility, and caution in our selection process. Otherwise, we may get hurt. Depending on how we handle the selection of habits, we can either turn out to be our own best friend or our worst enemy. The choice is ours to make.

We accumulate thousands of habits in our lifetime. Habits are necessary to our survival; we could not function without them. Here's the big question: what force drives us to choose one habit over another? I do not think there is a simple answer. Obviously, if we were not attracted to an activity in the first place, we would never proceed through the grueling process of converting that activity into an acquired habit. To capture our attention, it must appeal to our intellect as well as our emotions.

There are three memory banks, one assigned to each division of the mind. The entire Instinctual Division acts like a giant, long-term memory bank. Primary habits by definition are formed in a mysterious fashion and deposited in the Instinctual Division during the developmental stages of an organism. There is no way to figure out how, when, or where these original primary instincts formed. They come to us by birth for us to use wisely.

Acquired habits are formed in the Intellectual Division and are then transferred to the Instinctual Division as images. The memory bank of the Intellectual Division is dynamic and volatile and experiences constant shifts. The messages in this memory bank have a short life span. Frequent reinforcement is needed to retain the messages in this memory bank for longer than the usual period of time. The messages in this bank have two options:

either they are expelled completely or they are converted into biological memory chips, screened through the Emotional Division and imprinted in the Instinctual Division. This concept is extremely important in our learning process, because emotional balance will keep the pathway open for the transportation of the memory chip from the Intellectual Division to the Instinctual Division. This is one of many reasons people learn faster when they are emotionally stable.

Acquired habit formation occurs in three stages: (1) assimilation and analysis, (2) consolidation, and (3) transportation and imprinting.

STAGE 1: ASSIMILATION AND ANALYSIS

This stage commences as soon as you come into contact with the concept around which a habit will be formed. Let's take as an example learning to ride a bicycle. This is an activity that has captured most of our imaginations at one time in our lives. You want to learn to ride a bike, and you hop on board, determined to keep the vehicle upright. However, in the beginning you discover that balancing the bike against gravity is not very easy. If you lean too far to the right, you have to quickly adjust to the left or you'll topple over. Through trial and error you eventually learn to balance the bike.

All the while, your Intellectual Division is absorbing and analyzing the information in order to calculate the perfect formula to balance against gravity. In due course, your Intellectual Division develops a prototype of a synchronized response pattern that various parts of the body must follow. Once the Intellectual Division believes that it has perfected the formula, it will proceed to the next stage of consolidating all of the data it has collected into a memory chip.

STAGE 2: CONSOLIDATION

During this stage the intellect amalgamates all the knowledge obtained in the first stage, to create a permanent memory chip for riding a bicycle.

STAGE 3: TRANSPORTATION AND IMPRINTING

Once a complete memory chip of the activity is formed, you cannot afford to let it evaporate from your mind. The Intellectual Division's memory bank can only accommodate the image for a short amount of time. Without the third stage, the memory chip will eventually be dislodged and pushed out by newly acquired information. Therefore, the memory chip is transported to the Instinctual Division and imprinted as a habit so that it will stay with you on some level. If you do not ride a bike for twenty years, you may be a little wobbly when you first get on a bicycle again. But within a short period you'll pick it up as before, without having to go through the learning process all over again.

Some habits are more firmly imprinted than others. Motor coordination habits are usually the strongest, because there is little variation. Language skills are more complicated. For example, you may learn a foreign language in high school, but if you never use it again, it will be weakly imprinted and ultimately forgotten.

Age plays an important role in the strength of a habit's imprint. The younger you are, the stronger the imprint. Children

Approximate Life Span of an Idle, Nonaddictive Habit in the Instinctual Division

(based on more than 20 years of observational research)

TYPE OF HABIT	ACTIVE SHELF LIFE	SLOW DISINTEGRATION PHASE	RAPID DISINTEGRATION PHASE
Mother tongue (primary language)	15 years	20 years	5 years
Second language (acquired at a young age)	10 years	10 years	3 years
Tertiary language (acquired during adolescence)	5 years	3 years	2 years
Bicycle riding	25 years	20 years	10 years
Automobile driving	20 years	15 years	5 years
Typing	10 years	5 years	3 years
Tennis	5 years	3 years	1 year
In-line skating and ice-skating	5 years	3 years	2 years
Golf	3 years	2 years	1 year
Swimming	20 years	10 years	5 years
Gymnastics	5 years	3 years	2 years

TYPE OF HABIT	ACTIVE SHELF LIFE	SLOW DISINTEGRATION PHASE	RAPID DISINTEGRATION PHASE
Skiing	10 years	5 years	3 years
Knitting and sewing	10 years	5 years	3 years
Musical instrument	10 years	5 years	2 years
Trade (carpentry, welding, plumbing)	20 years	10 years	5 years
Painting and sculpting	10 years	5 years	3 years

are open to learning and have few distractions. That is why a very young child can learn to swim easily, while an adult will struggle with all of the fears accumulated over a lifetime.

Let's take language as an example. If you do not use a language for a long period of time, your memory of it will go into hibernation. However, traces of the memory chip of the language will be retained in both the Intellectual and Instinctual divisions of your mind. The traces of images in the Instinctual Division will remain for longer periods than those in the memory bank of the Intellectual Division. Eventually, if you continue not to use the language, the traces in the Instinctual Division will be partially obliterated and totally removed from the memory bank of the Intellectual Division.

There is a slight variation for habits involving motor coordination. For example, mechanically oriented habits such as skating, bicycle riding, or swimming take a long time to evaporate from the memory bank of the Intellectual Division, and even longer to evaporate just partially from the memory bank of the Instinctual Division. Once a person learns to swim, ride a bicycle, or drive a car, he can never forget the basics of these activities, as they are imprinted in the memory bank of the Instinctual Division. But acrobatic moves associated with activities such as fancy diving, or tricks on a bicycle, as we see performed in the circus, disappear fast, unless they are reinforced frequently.

Unlike motor skills, language skills need more frequent reinforcements to be retained in the memory bank of both the Intellectual Division and the Instinctual Division. The mother tongue is the only exception to this rule—the reason being, the strong emotional attachment and sense of identity associated with it. We know that it is not easy to forget the first language we learn, even after not using it for decades.

The memory bank assigned to the Emotional Division is relatively stable and less likely to experience shifts. Activities imprinted in the Intellectual Division, such as typing or bicycle riding, will not register there; but activities that evoke emotional responses, such as touching a hot plate, will be strongly imprinted in the memory bank of the Emotional Division. The depth of imprinting depends upon the strength of the emotional response. If the plate is red hot, it will elicit a strong response from the pain center and have a deeper imprinting in the memory bank of the Emotional Division. The psychological component of the event remains intact in the emotions, making it an unforgettable experience. However, the physical component of the actual event is forgotten within a short period of time.

On the other hand, activities such as smoking, drinking alcohol, or engaging in sex evoke an attractive, pleasant, comfortable experience in the Emotional Division, which in turn is stored as images of pleasure-releasing activities in the memory bank. Just as a painful experience repels a person away from a particular activity, a pleasurable experience lures a person toward it. But the difference in the case of a pleasurable activity is that a person is more likely to become preoccupied with that activity, and thereby develop a habit. Once an image of the activity is fully engraved in the memory bank of the Emotional Division, it is extremely difficult to get rid of that memory chip. This applies to activities that evoke either pleasure or pain.

Unfortunately, most of us take habit formation for granted. A person with good habits will pay little attention to them, since they don't harm him. But this person can actually further enhance his good habits by obtaining a better understanding of habit formation. On the other hand, not all habits serve us well and guard our interests. If a person cultivates a bad and sometimes dangerous habit, it could potentially ruin his life. On any given day there is a possibility of turning an innocent, incidental activity into a well-established, and not so desirable, habit such as smoking.

In the beginning, many people feel that a casual acquaintance with certain activities will not hurt them. They are associating with these activities for the purpose of a onetime pleasurable experience. They fail to realize that an activity that can elicit a positive and appealing response from their emotions may compel them to repeat such an activity numerous times. Unknowingly, these individuals become compulsive slaves to that activity.

Developing an Addictive Habit

What distinguishes the person who throws caution and cultural mores to the wind and engages in addictive behaviors, such as smoking, even at the risk of ostracism, disease, and death, from the person who does not? The personality traits and mental disposition of addicts will eventually determine the course of their bondage. Often the initial motivation of the person who later becomes addicted is curiosity or rebellion. A young person may sneak a cigarette to assert independence or because he wonders what it's like. But it is what happens next that determines whether he will develop a passion for smoking or walk away.

Since none of us is born with addictive habits, and they are not necessary for our survival, how do they become entrenched? Modern behavioral scientists have provided many clues to the course of addiction—such as an individual's inherent affinity for a particular addictive habit, personality traits, socioeconomic status, educational background, cultural views, and, finally, the nature of the addictive habit itself. Genetic factors are known to play a role in a person's affinity for a particular addictive habit.

Tendencies are not inevitabilities, however, and socioeconomic factors only go so far to explain addiction. By and large, exposure to an addictive habit ranks number one among various causative factors, but it certainly doesn't explain the mysterious origins and drives of addictive habits. Even those with all the odds against them do not necessarily become addicts. For a habit to form, the Emotional Division of the mind must first be primed to crave relief through addictive behavior. It must be provoked by an internal need—what I call an addictive drive. These drives include deprivation, entitlement, invincibility, disenchantment, insecurity, and defiance, and they will be described later in greater detail.

Let's take a closer look at how the smoking habit can develop. Usually between the ages of twelve and fifteen, an individual will experiment with smoking. The first attempt is always triggered by an external need, such as peer pressure, curiosity, stress, and the like. At first the individual will find the experience repulsive, but on subsequent attempts there will be some kind of elation with each drag, which will be registered in the Emotional Division. Thus the seed is planted. Seeking out the repetition of the pleasure, the Emotional Division will trigger subsequent smoking, and the activity is transformed from an external need to an internal need. In the course of time, the smoker won't even pay attention to the external factors that led to picking up the first cigarette. Before long, cigarettes become an integral part of the person's lifestyle.

Once the image of an addictive habit is lodged in the memory bank of the Emotional Division, it begins to expand its power base without any interruption from the Intellectual Division. Depending on the individual's tolerance, disposition, patience, attitude, outlook, and circumstances, the smoker will find that the influence of an addictive habit extends to the entire Emotional Division, which leads to a strong desire to associate with an addictive activity at all times, on all occasions. Boredom, nervousness, anxiety, anger, disappointment, and frustration demand the good taste and pleasure of a cigarette. The absence of the substance provokes strong cravings.

These cravings demand satisfaction, and the longer the Intellectual Division takes to comply with the demands of the Emotional Division, the stronger the intensity of the cravings. At one point, irrespective of its reasons for noncompliance, the

Intellectual Division will be forced by the Emotional Division to take immediate action. This fact will not be apparent until the Intellectual Division takes an opposing stand and tries to say no to smoking. Most smokers try at some point to contain or overcome their habit, only to find their cravings getting stronger as the addictive habit dispenses a strong signal to both the Intellectual Division and the Instinctual Division to pursue the activity. The nucleus of the smoking habit is internal and is well guarded by the Emotional Division from any outside interference.

Animals of a lower intellectual order have been provided with the requisite primary habits for survival, but they are less capable of learning from exposure to the environment. For example, birds migrate to the south in the winter months, because they are driven by their primary habits; the polar bear knows how to handle subzero temperatures through hibernation. But if human beings were to rely on their basic primary habits to survive in similar temperatures, they would end up as frozen Popsicles. Nature fine-tunes the behavior of animals—except that of human beings—through their primary habits. Because animals mainly operate through primary habits, with very little modification and manipulation from the Intellectual Division, their overall behavior is predictable and consistent with species-specific responses. In contrast, human beings have to rely more on their acquired habits than their primary habits for one reason: we are bestowed with a powerful intellect, a vivid imagination, and unlimited freedom to choose our way of life.

But the freedom we enjoy does not come cheap. Nature has warned us that we are held accountable for our actions and will be punished by nature if we misbehave. Furthermore, nature controls the type of punitive action and time frame for dispensing consequences. For example, everyone knows that we pay a heavy price for selecting bad habits such as smoking. Bad habits can inflict irrevocable damage on a person and bring misery not only to the individual involved but also to others in close association with that person. Unfortunately, nature refuses to listen to our explanations and excuses for selecting bad habits. It usually dispenses appropriate penalties for our misdeeds. We must endure the consequences of our own bad choices.

Most important, remember that once a habit is established, it is impossible to erase the image from the mind. At best, we can tame the influence of an unwanted habit. We have to expend a lot of energy, effort, and time to manifest a small victory over an entrenched, unwanted bad habit. Because we rely more on our acquired habits for survival, what we learn has a major impact on our behavior and existence.

Based on my observation of different characteristics of all addictive habits, I have classified them into three primary categories:

- Mind-soothing addictive habits
- Mind-altering addictive habits
- Mind-provoking addictive habits

MIND-SOOTHING ADDICTIVE HABITS

Cigarette smoking, drinking coffee or tea, compulsive eating, and compulsive sex fall into this category. The comforting and soothing effects of these activities captivate the attention of participants and tie them to these habits. The unique feature of these habits is that they allow the mental status to remain intact. For instance, a cigarette smoker does not lose mental balance like an alcoholic. The dangers that accompany these habits are well hidden, and thus they appear harmless. It is not easy for the individual to identify and acknowledge the harmful effects of these habits even after years of associating with them. By providing a false sense of security, these habits con the individual into remaining loyal for years. For instance, even after decades of aggressive campaigning against the smoking habit because of health hazards, millions of people all over the world still smoke without any reservation.

MIND-ALTERING ADDICTIVE HABITS

Some of the most notorious, mind-crippling, and unhealthy habits belong to this group. They include alcohol and various drugs. All of these habits are based on chemical-substance abuse of one type or other. Besides providing the expected comfort, euphoria, ecstasy, and thrill, the addictive chemical substances affect and alter the mental status to a lesser or greater degree. People who are involved with these habits experience temporary or permanent impairment of memory, mental balance, reasoning, judgment, and physical reflexes. These habits adversely affect an individual physically, mentally, and spiritually. Eventually, addicts may end up as mental cripples and physical invalids. The substances that are incriminated with these habits range from "soft" drugs such as alcohol, Valium, codeine, and marijuana, to "hard drugs" such as cocaine, crack, heroin, PCP, and methamphetamines.

MIND-PROVOKING ADDICTIVE HABITS

There are certain issues about a human being that one can spend centuries trying to explain in logical terms, but they will still remain a mystery. Mind-provoking addictive habits are one such entity. Typical examples of mind-provoking addictions are gambling and the lust for power and wealth. A compulsive gambler cannot stop gambling even if he is on a winning streak, since his expectations are limitless. On the other hand, if he loses, he continues to play to make up for his losses. Win or lose, the mind-provoking addiction will not give an individual the needed gratification and satisfaction to release him from its stranglehold. Despite the absence of physical mediating agents, these addictions are extremely powerful and will not let a person go without sapping his spirits, hopes, and future. Eventually he ends up restless, agitated, sleepless, and preoccupied with his addiction just like a cocaine, crack, or heroin addict.

The striking feature of mind-provoking addictive habits is that there is no physical mediating agent (e.g., alcohol, cigarettes, food) to trigger a chemical response. There is no tangible explanation for the power of these habits. Rather, people are hooked on an "idea." For example, some people are hooked on the idea of basking in unlimited wealth and power, which is the basis of this type of addiction. The persistent idea keeps these addicts running in circles because their target is an unreachable goal. Not realizing this fact, they embark on a never-ending journey into oblivion. The insatiable desire to reach their goal at any cost provokes these addicts to concoct extraordinary measures and to implement them without fail. The actions they undertake without knowing what the outcome could be give these people a greater thrill than actually reaching their destination. The euphoria and the thrill hidden in the actions they take keep them going forever, and, believe it or not, these addicts cannot get off this roller coaster ride.

Bad Habits Die Hard

Many therapies attempt to treat compulsive behaviors and addictions by altering a person's brain chemistry. But you cannot treat the *mind* through the *brain*. As we have seen, the mind has its own distinctive characteristics and a different set of rules. The choice to adopt a habit—and make no mistake about it, it *is* a choice—takes place in the mind. This is a critical point, because our habits can make or break us. A habit can be friend or foe, and it is the mind's charge to be vigilant, to understand the consequences of the habits we adopt. Once a "bad" habit takes hold in the mind, it locks into place, and the emotional resistance to giving it up is ferocious.

Most people don't realize the tenacity of their habit until the first time they try to walk away from it. They tell themselves they can give up the habit any time they want; it only requires self-control. They rarely consider themselves addicts—especially when their behaviors don't visibly interfere with the daily workings of their lives. Desperation only sets in after they repeatedly fail to stop. The habit defies everything they believe about their intelligence and interior strength. It shakes their confidence to the core.

Because the nucleus of a habit is the drive or the compulsion to associate with that habit, the compulsion is deeply entrenched in the mind. For instance, an individual attempting to give up smoking will usually focus on the number of cigarettes he smokes, or the type—low-tar, filtered, and the like. These are external factors, completely incidental to overcoming the habit. The compulsion to smoke is deeply embedded in the mind. It is invisible and intangible. You can't visualize it with a CT scan or an MRI. You can't capture it in a blood test. Yet there it is—a formidable foe.

THE DRIVE TO SMOKE

Tom, a thirty-six-year-old investment banker, came to me for help in stopping smoking. He was married to a smoker—a red flag, because when a spouse is also a smoker and is not willing to stop, it is naturally hard on the person who does want to quit.

I asked Tom to tell me about himself and to try to identify his reasons for smoking. As he spoke, a picture emerged of an intense, goal-oriented individual with an overwhelming desire to succeed at work. I also saw a man who was very sensitive and sentimental, with a touch of insecurity and low self-esteem. He hated deadlines and uncertainties in life.

Tom's father was also an investment banker, involved in mergers and acquisitions. He was extremely successful, and from a very young age Tom tried to emulate his father in every way possible in order to win his approval. As a result, Tom was always in some sort of emotional upheaval. As he had never tried to be himself, he had never been at peace and truly contented. He used his smoking habit to calm down, boost his confidence, improve his concentration, and relax after a long day's work.

In 1998 Tom decided to stop smoking. The habit was beginning to drain him of energy, and he'd suffered several severe bronchial infections. He didn't believe he'd be able to stop cold turkey, so he decided to use a nicotine patch. For the first few days, he was reasonably comfortable without cigarettes. But after two months he realized that he was less comfortable with not smoking than he'd been in the early days—just the opposite of what he'd expected. He was more irritable, and he'd started to bite his nails and overeat out of nervousness. He also felt that

(continued)

he was not as effective at work. He began to fret. "I have a high-pressure job," he said. "I can't afford to slack off."

One day, about five months after he had quit smoking, Tom was having a particularly awful day at work. Nothing was going right. His clients were making outrageous demands, his assistants were ineffective and were letting him down, and he felt that the world was closing in on him. He described the feeling as claustrophobic. At that moment, he pulled off the patch and ran down the stairs to the street, where he bummed a cigarette from a colleague. He lit it, took a deep drag, and immediately felt good and relieved, even though he was coughing. "I thought, what was the harm?" he said. "It wasn't such a bad deal to get so much relief from one cigarette. I didn't even smoke the whole thing. I went back in, reapplied the patch, and did pretty well for the rest of the day."

Tom didn't have another cigarette for eight days, and he was able to cope fairly easily. On the eighth day, he felt a "tug" from the smoking habit, and this time he didn't fight it. He pulled off the patch, went outside, and smoked two cigarettes before returning to his office.

Within four weeks of his first puff, he was smoking three or four cigarettes a day. As the days passed, he began to pick up the pace, and soon he was back to his usual one pack a day. He explained that he still used the patch as a supplementary tool whenever he had to go for long periods without smoking.

During the next few years, Tom tried to quit smoking several times, but he always failed. When he came to my office in 2004, he was desperate to stop but afraid he would not be able to overcome his smoking habit.

For Tom to be successful, he had to excise the pleasurable imprint that was firmly embedded in his mind. As you will see, the task requires a strategy well beyond slapping on a patch.

Part Two

The Prasad Method:
Mind over Habit

THE PROCESS OF QUITTING smoking is not for the faint of heart. There's no such thing as a magic fix. Life isn't easy, and it isn't supposed to be. I often have patients complain, "It wasn't supposed to be this way." Well, who said so? All you have to do is look at human history to know that life is a battleground, not a playground. The truth is, we are still struggling every day for our survival, just like our ancestors. Even with the best planning and most conscientious effort, things don't always work out as we wish. However, we do have a lot of control over the quality of our lives and the way we choose to use our God-given talents and opportunities during our short stay on earth. To stop smoking, you must take personal responsibility for your plight, and reject excuses and sense of victimization.

It's not enough to know smoking is bad for you. You must believe it. The fact is, people act on what they *believe,* not what they *know.* The difference between what you know and what you believe is the real disparity between the action you should take and the action you do take. When we keep our ears open, we hear lots of sensible advice and compelling information. Why doesn't this information transfer to our beliefs? The information we hear has to pass through an emotional screen composed of our likes and dislikes. When we hear information that appeals to us, it receives easy passage. On the other hand, when we hear information that is not to our liking, it must pass through many more barriers. What we know for a fact is registered in the Intellectual Division. What we believe is registered in our Emotional Division.

Every smoker knows that cigarettes are not in his best interest, but until this knowledge becomes a part of his belief system, any attempt to quit lacks real teeth. A smoker may want to quit, but when push comes to shove he does not really want to part with the comfort and pleasure he derives from smoking. He may try to cut corners and smoke only a couple of cigarettes a day, but ultimately he will fail.

When a patient sits across from me in my office, I help show the difference between the two and work toward narrowing the gap. I present it this way: "Let's say you believe you've become allergic to nicotine. The next puff will kill you. There is no room for error. Would you smoke?"

"Of course not" is the inevitable response. In this case the imminent visceral threat is capable of altering the belief system. Fear for survival immediately collapses the wall between the intellect and the emotions. Short of such a threat, the emotions are reluctant to give up the pleasure. They coax the smoker to overlook the threats and mitigate against them. A person's belief system must be altered in order to convince him to take actions that are not pleasing.

How do we know the truth? When it comes to beliefs, human beings are skillful at twisting the actual truth to their own version of the truth. We see this phenomenon all around us every day—in politics, advertising, business, and religious practices.

Walter was a distinguished fifty-two-year-old professor of world politics at a leading university. He had been toying with the idea of quitting smoking for about ten years but only became serious when he felt his health was deteriorating. When he came to me, he said he often felt exhausted and had frequent bouts of bronchitis. He readily attributed these symptoms to smoking, yet he had been unable to stop. He'd tried the patch, Nicorette gum, and the smoking-cessation medication Zyban. None of his attempts were successful.

"I cannot understand the stranglehold that smoking has over me," he told me. "I am certainly intelligent. I am also disciplined and diligent. Yet in this one area I have failed miserably. Why?"

To get to the bottom of the question, I asked Walter to talk about himself and tell me about his life. He described a Bohemian background. His parents were from Eastern Europe, and when Walter was a child he spent a lot of time in Europe. He loved and admired his five uncles there. All of them were intellectuals. They were also chain-smokers. Walter started smoking when he was twelve years old, and he smoked a pack a day by the time he was fifteen. When Walter was a teenager, he participated in many demonstrations against Communist rule while visiting his extended family in Eastern Europe. He often saw NO SMOKING signs in public places, and they were in Russian. He and his friends delighted in smoking right underneath these signs as an expression of defiance.

In present times, Walter noted that he especially admired two professors at the university who had written many highly acclaimed books. One was nominated for a Nobel Prize. Both of them were chain-smokers.

On a deeply emotional level, Walter had a great deal of admiration for smoking. He believed cigarettes were associated with the intelligentsia and were a symbol of freedom. On some level, Walter believed his essential personality and his creative abilities were tied to his smoking habit. He feared that without cigarettes he would lose his intellectual and professional edge.

Without realizing it, Walter had allowed the world around him to shape his perception, beliefs, and behavior, thus letting cigarettes have a dominant influence over him. I told Walter that by giving cigarettes the credit for his creativity and performance, he was insulting his Maker and the entire human race. "If cigarettes can produce Nobel Prize winners out of dummies, why isn't the world full of geniuses?" I asked. "You were born with a powerful brain. Cigarettes cannot enhance your brain power. On the contrary, lack of oxygen and increases in carbon dioxide and carbon monoxide can lower your brain power."

This hit the nail on the head for Walter. Now he was not scared to give up smoking. He now believed that smoking would harm his brain power, not improve it. He believed in himself, not in cigarettes anymore. Today he is a comfortable nonsmoker.

If you fight against nature's truth, you will lead a life of suffering. People say, "I love the truth . . . as long as it works out for me." Nature's truth is another matter. It is black and white. We want to negotiate the shades of gray. However, our excuses and explanations are all a waste of time. Nature doesn't care why you can't stop smoking. Nature sees only the action and passes judgment accordingly.

We are imperfect creatures. We make mistakes. But know this: every mistake you make carries a price. If you smoke cigarettes, you will have limited lung capacity and your life will be shortened. Nature does not take into consideration your special circumstances. There are no free passes.

To stop smoking, you must follow these steps:

Step 1: Understand Why You Must Quit. In order to successfully quit smoking, you must be uncomfortable with your habit. Obviously, as long as you are comfortable, you have little motivation to change. But something converts the comfortable habit into the uncomfortable habit—health issues, family problems, professional or social interferences, spiritual issues, legal complications, and so on.

You must want to break the habit. You can no longer bear the idea of continuing. You may try to give up the habit but fail repeatedly. The desire to break the habit grows into a firm resolve or commitment to become permanently and happily free of it.

Step 2: Determine the Depth of Your Addiction. The more information you have about your enemy, the easier it is to conquer. Knowing your own strengths and weaknesses will give you an edge in the manner of your response to the difficulties of quitting.

Step 3: Identify Your Addictive Profile. You must know why you smoke. What are the emotional triggers of your addiction? I have defined six primary triggers of the smoking habit: deprivation, entitlement, invincibility, disenchantment, insecurity, and defiance. The Addictive Profile, which is formed by one or more of these drives, is the engine that charges up addictive behavior.

Step 4: Make the Break. Make the leap from the last puff to no puff. The best way to quit is to pick a time and place to terminate the habit in one shot. This method enables you to pool all your strength to inflict a mortal blow on your enemy in a single stroke.

Step 5: Become a Comfortable Nonsmoker. Your final goal should be to change from being an uncomfortable, disheartened smoker to being a comfortable, permanent, and proud nonsmoker.

Step 6: Eliminate the Mentality of Addiction. You bring closure to the habit and move on to lead a life happily free of its constraints.

STEP 1

Understand Why You Must Quit

RICK, THE PROMINENT CEO of a major organization, came to see me three years ago to help him stop smoking. During our initial consultation he explained that six months earlier, he, his secretary, and one of his assistants had decided to kick the habit together. All three felt that it was time to say good-bye to cigarettes. They focused on four reasons: (1) health, (2) inconvenience, (3) expense, and (4) negative image—although the order of importance was different for each of them. They agreed to quit cold turkey and made a pact to encourage and support one another in their efforts.

Rick's secretary eventually quit smoking with considerable hardship. At one point it was touch and go. His assistant had an easier time. From the first day, Rick himself was confident that he'd make it. However, to his surprise and chagrin, he failed miserably. He could not survive more than two days without cigarettes, and those two days were hell. Finally, on the third day, he decided he'd just smoke two or three cigarettes a day. For a few days Rick pretended he was making progress, but after three weeks he had to admit that he'd failed.

Rick just couldn't understand the outcome. He'd expected to have an easier time than the other two. After all, he'd never smoked more than a pack a day, whereas his secretary had smoked two and a half packs, and his assistant had smoked two packs. Furthermore, Rick had always considered himself highly disciplined. He thought about it, worked up his nerve, and several weeks later made another attempt to quit. That failed, too, as did a third try.

Finally, Rick had to acknowledge that he was facing a formidable enemy. He was a proud man, and this habit really humiliated him. He was desperate to stop smoking, if only to prove to himself that he could really do it. Otherwise, he could not live with himself. When he sat in my office, Rick asked me if I had an explanation for why he'd failed to quit smoking, while his secretary and assistant had succeeded.

Rick's secretary felt that the smoking habit was getting too expensive, and it was also just too inconvenient. If she wanted a cigarette, she had to take the elevator down to the street outside the office building. She also wanted to succeed to gain Rick's admiration, although this reason was less effective as a motivator. Since she was in reasonably good health, her motivation wasn't strongly health related. She succeeded in quitting, but she had a hard time.

Rick's assistant had undergone quadruple bypass the previous year, and he knew his days were numbered if he didn't quit. He was already feeling short of breath. He had worked hard all his life to reach the pinnacle of his career. He wasn't about to throw it all away over cigarettes. He quit with relative ease.

From the beginning, Rick underestimated his enemy. His motivation to quit smoking was weak. Expense didn't bother him. Inconvenience wasn't an issue; he could smoke in his private office whenever he wanted. He was in good health. Smoking didn't really have a notably negative effect. These factors added up to a sense of invincibility. Deep down, Rick didn't believe that smoking would hurt him. Besides, he enjoyed his cigarettes, especially in the morning with his coffee and after work when he relaxed. He figured he was entitled to this one small pleasure. He was a hard worker, and a good husband and father. He felt entitled. After trying and failing to quit several times, he was starting to feel insecure. He wondered if he could do it. Insecurity can be something of a vicious circle, which continues to feed the failure. Rick needed to acknowledge and attack his emotional reactions before he could succeed.

Rick had not yet experienced his moment of truth. Simply put, the moment of truth comes when the habit that once provided such relief is no longer comfortable.

Discovering Your Moment of Truth: An Inside-Out Approach

The following process is a variation of the one I use with my patients to help them realize their moment of truth and help them come to their own understanding of why they must quit smoking. It is designed to help you literally *change your mind* about smoking. By coming to the realization of why you really need to quit and by understanding why you started smoking in the first place, you can make up your mind to become a comfortable nonsmoker who isn't sorry to put a habit behind them.

Know Why You Want to Quit

The first question I ask people who come to me to stop smoking is this: "Why have you decided to launch a personal vendetta against your beloved friend and companion?" That gets their attention!

I admire the people who come to my office to stop smoking. They usually arrive filled with enthusiasm and determination to complete their missions. In buoyant voices, they talk about how eager they are to get the nasty smoking habit out of their lives, and they have dozens of reasons to do so. However, I am only interested in the reason that has firmly captivated their attention and compelled them to take action. I want to know about the force that drives them to forsake their old friend and companion—the cigarette. It takes a powerful motivation to succeed at this challenge. That motivation must come from within, and it must withstand the test of time.

If you look around you, it may seem obvious why someone should wish to quit smoking. Today society has taken a dim view of the smoker and his habit. People have grown intolerant of the smoke spewing into the air and the stench it emits. Most people consider smoking to be a dirty habit. A person who smokes in public cannot help noticing the disapproving glares from those around him. Laws forbid smoking in restaurants and offices, and the hapless smoker is relegated to designated places. These advances are important ways to curb the smoking habit in society, but they cause great bitterness among smokers, who view them as coercive. Coercion, even to advance a noble cause, never works as a solution on a personal level. If guilt is the driving force, there is no chance that people will permanently give up the habit. The only effective motivation is an internal, voluntary desire to protect and preserve your quality of life by eliminating the poisonous bonds of the smoking habit.

For example, Jenna, a twenty-year-old woman, came to my office to stop her four-year smoking habit. She told me that she was committed to succeed, no matter what it took. When I asked her the reason she was committed to stopping, she said that she was very much in love with a man who despised smoking, and she needed to stop to show him she was serious about the relationship. I immediately told her it wouldn't work. "You can't stop for someone else," I said. When I refused to take her as my patient, she was furious and stormed out of my office.

Six years later, I saw Jenna again. She told me she'd gone to a hypnotist when I'd previously rejected her, and she had stopped smoking for three months. Then one day she had a fight with her boyfriend and, in a fit of rage, she went back to smoking. I wasn't surprised. In order to succeed, it was essential that she believe from her mind, heart, and soul that smoking was not in her best interest. You can't stop smoking as a favor to another person.

I also believe that you cannot be successful if you are a comfortable smoker. Yes, there are a few of those. You have to be uncomfortable with your habit. The strong desire to quit must engage every one of your senses. It must be internal, not external. For example, an external reason for quitting might be, "My husband can't stand my smoking." An internal reason is, "I can't stand the discomfort of smoking."

Addiction is not an external reality, but an internal one, which must be viewed from the inside out. Unless you fully understand yourself and your motivations, you have no hope of permanently releasing yourself from the habit. If you've tried to overcome your habit before, only to fail, this time you'll start from an entirely different place. Instead of trying to wrestle the cigarette to the ground and kill it, begin by ignoring the substance altogether. Focus instead on yourself. No two addicts are alike. Their temperament, outlook, attitude, priorities, expectations, and limitations are different from those of every other addict. For this reason, only *you* can break your habit. Not your doctor, not a pill, not your husband, or therapist, or support group. Just you.

THE RIGHT WAY: THE INSIDE-OUT APPROACH	THE WRONG WAY: THE OUTSIDE-IN APPROACH
Don't talk. Commit yourself.	Keep talking about giving up smoking.
Don't try to stop. Just stop.	Say you "would like" to quit.
Believe smoking is not good for you.	Promise to give it a good try.
Stop smoking for yourself—to improve your quality of life.	Decide to stop to please your spouse or boss.
Rely on your patience, tolerance, and strength to defeat the discomfort.	Rely on the patch, gum, or other crutches.
Prepare to tackle the immediate changes to your routine from the last puff to no puff.	Change your brand, cut down, or otherwise try to wean yourself from cigarettes.
Make it your goal to put cigarettes out of mind, not just out of sight.	Get rid of all visible signs of smoking—ashtrays, lighters, etc. Stay away from smokers so you won't be tempted.

The hardships you are encountering are mainly due to your own choices. You're responsible for your predicament, and you must spearhead the campaign to save yourself. This job cannot be delegated.

The reason you decide to quit also needs to be permanent—not something you do for a short period of time, like only while you are pregnant. My patient Marilyn was a thirty-two-year-old mother who wanted to quit smoking. During our initial conversation, she disclosed that three years ago she had given up smoking for ten months and then had gone back to smoking. Naturally, I was curious to know why she started to smoke again after such a long interval. She replied that she had given up smoking on her own during the first month of pregnancy. By the ninth month, she had forgotten all about cigarettes. For reasons unbeknownst to her, she started to think about smoking a month after the delivery. A few days later, she wanted to have just one cigarette for old times' sake. One drag was all she needed to reestablish her smoking habit. Her pregnancy was a short-term reason to withhold the habit temporarily, and she had programmed her mind not to think about cigarettes for that particular duration. Once she delivered her child, the compelling motivation was gone.

Many of my patients tell me that they plan to clean their houses completely and get rid of all ashtrays and other smoking paraphernalia before they quit, and they're quite surprised when I don't express immediate approval of this plan. As one man put it, "Out of sight, out of mind. Right, Doc?"

Not at all! In reality, getting rid of all the vestiges of the habit doesn't really help the cause. It's just another external approach to an internal problem. As long as the addictive drives are intact, a smoker will crave a cigarette even if he is on a desert island without his stash. It is the craving to smoke, not the availability of smoking paraphernalia, that's the issue here.

If you're about to stop smoking but are scared of your enemy, if you feel almost certain that you'll fail in its presence, you've already lost the battle before you've even begun. Conversely, if you have taken an inside-out approach, and are ready to put cigarettes out of your mind, even when they are not out of your sight, you will win the battle.

Understand Why You Started Smoking

Keep in mind the reason why you originally started smoking is equally, if not more, important than the reason you continue to smoke. For example, a teenager may start smoking cigarettes or drinking alcohol to establish his adulthood and to spite his elders. The anger, bitterness, and rebellious elements of this teenager will be incorporated as an integral part of the habit. Years later, that individual might have forgotten about all his teenage shenanigans, but he cannot expect the addictive habit to erase these issues from its memory bank. The habit may even use them against the individual at the time of his struggle to part with the habit. In this instance, the smoking habit makes you feel that by giving up smoking, you are actually parting with your individuality and self-identity.

In such cases, it is possible that immediately after giving up smoking, anger or bitterness dominates the emotional disposition of the individual. I have come across this kind of reaction in the past, and I warn my patients in advance of such unexpected outbursts and prepare them to deal with them. Isn't it amazing that what started out as a simple, silly, childhood bizarre behavior years ago can weave a complex, formidable obstacle for his progress at a later date?

I help my patients move toward a fuller understanding of self. One's identity should not be based on external features and behaviors, such as skin color, clothing style, profession, zip code, the type of food you eat, club memberships, the language you speak, house of worship, whether you drink alcohol, whether you smoke, and the like. These factors are shallow. They may show style but they offer no substance to a well-formed sense of identity. When you rely on external factors, you are actually allowing the world to define you instead of taking a stand on your own. On the other hand, if you try to define yourself based on sound internal factors—your values, talents, priorities, temperament, expectations, tolerance, and life goals—you set yourself on a noble path. You become determined to reach your goals, even if it's hard to do. You can focus on the journey of your life without being bothered by insignificant or unproductive distractions.

Commit to Becoming a Comfortable Nonsmoker

State your commitment in irrevocable terms. When questioned, people will often say, "I'd like to stop smoking." This is not a commitment, only a wish. There is a big difference between wishful thinking and commitment. Wishful thinking leads a person to give it a good try; when he fails, he will then say, "Better luck next time." When there is true commitment, failure is not an option.

Think of it as a contract you are making with yourself that has no escape clause. To be successful, the contract must include:

- A decision to tackle the habit on its terms and conditions, not those you imagine or invent
- A decision that failure is not an option
- A decision to be not just free of the habit but *comfortable* and *productive* without it
- A decision that you, not your habit, will decide your fate

EVALUATE YOUR REASONS FOR QUITTING

Sit down and seriously think about all the reasons you have for quitting smoking. Place each of the reasons why you want to quit smoking into either the Internal box or the External box in the blank table below. Calculate your score at the end. It will become part of your total Smoking Cessation Struggle Index—that is, the relative difficulty you will have breaking the habit.

EXTERNAL REASONS INCLUDE:
- My doctor, spouse, and friends tell me smoking is bad for me.
- Smoking is inconvenient and expensive.
- I don't like being treated like a pariah because I smoke.
- I want to impress others.
- I want to set an example for my children.

INTERNAL REASONS INCLUDE:
- I believe smoking is not in my best interest.
- I want to have this monkey off my back.

- I want to feel good about myself and believe in myself.
- I will no longer be a slave to this habit.

EXTERNAL REASONS TO QUIT	INTERNAL REASONS TO QUIT
1. _____	1. _____
2. _____	2. _____
3. _____	3. _____
4. _____	4. _____
5. _____	5. _____

Score: For each External reason, give yourself 4 points. For each Internal reason, give yourself −1 point.
Total your score: _____
Enter the result in the Smoking Cessation Struggle Index calculator on page 111.

STEP 2

Determine the Depth of Your Addiction

THE NEXT STEP is to get practical. Name your poison. Each habit has unique characteristics that must be thoroughly understood in order to wage a successful fight. To conquer the enemy, you must understand your enemy. What is your personal association with smoking? When did you start the habit? What pleasurable associations does it have? How much do you smoke, and which cigarettes do you enjoy the most? Being able to answer these questions is empowering. It takes the mystery out of your habit so you can conquer it. Let's look at each aspect of your habit individually. Don't be discouraged if you find yourself among the hard cases. The fact that it may be tougher for you to quit than for your friend whose habit is less entrenched only means you will have to use smarter strategies to defeat this wily enemy. These strategies will be provided in the next section. For now, just concentrate on the objective elements of your habit. Be as accurate as possible. It might help to use a notebook to write down your answers.

THE AGE YOU STARTED SMOKING

With few exceptions, most people are introduced to smoking in their midteens. Teenagers fall into the trap of this habit when they want to be accepted by their peers. Being impulsive, inquisitive, and adventurous, they are open to trying something new. Teenagers also smoke to declare their freedom and defiance of the "system." The younger the age when you start smoking, the stronger the imprint of the habit in the Emotional Division, making it much harder to give up. If you started smoking during your teen years, it will be especially difficult to quit.

Sam, forty years old, wanted to give up his smoking habit. At an intellectual level, he was absolutely clear about the dangers of smoking, and he knew it was in his best interest to quit for good. He had tried many times to stop, but he consistently hit some kind of an obstacle that prevented him from succeeding. As we talked about his life, it became apparent to me that deep down in his Emotional Division, Sam harbored an idyllic image of smoking based on his youthful impressions. Both of his parents were educated and professional businesspeople. When he was young, he had witnessed their coming home from work dead tired and cranky. As soon as they freshened up, they relaxed in the family room with a glass of wine and cigarettes. Sam could still recall the scent of the warm smoke as it wafted into the air and the way his parents would sigh with relief as they began to unwind. A cigarette could wipe away the cares of the day. When his parents entertained, Sam also noticed that the smokers always seemed to have more fun than everyone else in the room. The image was firmly imprinted in Sam's mind as he equated smoking with relaxation. He was unconsciously convinced that if he gave up cigarettes, he would be tense and cranky.

The age you are when you first try to quit smoking also plays a crucial role in success. Teenagers who haven't been smoking for very long will have a difficult time trying to quit smoking. The intellect of a youngster is not mature enough to process messages from the environment in the proper context, making it much easier for the wrong impressions to be formed in the mind. The distorted impressions, firmly planted in the mind, make the fight against the smoking habit a real uphill battle.

On the other end of the spectrum, older smokers often don't see a point in giving up a habit toward the end of their lifetime. Richard was sixty-five years old, hardy looking and gruff. He announced that he wanted to give up his smoking habit. He had smoked two packs of cigarettes a day for fifty years. He suffered from a chronic cough and was highly motivated to stop. When he came to see me, Richard said that he had recently retired as a field-worker for the telephone company, and he was looking forward to a wonderful retired life with his wife. I felt that everything was in his favor, as Richard was mature, ready, and willing, and had a strong reason to stop smoking. I thought he would give up smoking without any problems. I was wrong. Richard struggled much harder than most of my patients. At one point I was about to give up on him. In the end it took an extreme effort over the course of almost a year for Richard to succeed.

Over time, I began to notice similar difficulties from patients over age sixty. Why did they have such a hard time quitting? I finally determined that these patients had an underlying barrier that they weren't even aware of. They regarded their time on earth as short, and didn't really believe that quitting would matter. In Richard's case, this difficulty was exacerbated by boredom. He had too much time on his hands. I suggested he start volunteering at the gift shop in his local hospital, and he found it immensely rewarding. If you are in Richard's position, take some time to consider your self-story and the need to value every day. It will make your effort to quit smoking less of a struggle.

The Type of Cigarette You Smoke

There are three major types of cigarettes—regular nonfiltered, regular filtered, and mentholated filtered. Both filters and menthol influence the pleasure derived by the smoker. Smokers have stated that there is a significant reduction in the level of satisfaction when they switch from nonfiltered to filtered cigarettes. Even though a relatively small percentage of smokers choose mentholated brands, these smokers experience more problems giving up cigarettes than those who smoke regular brands. If you smoke mentholated cigarettes, you might consider switching to regular in the weeks before you quit.

The Number of Cigarettes You Smoke

The actual number of cigarettes you smoke every day defines the depth of your dependence. The rule of thumb is that the hardship encountered in quitting is directly proportional to the number of cigarettes smoked.

When You Smoke Your First Cigarette of the Day

The first cigarette of the day is the best and most satisfying cigarette of all. Every smoker likes the first cigarette, but not all attempt to smoke as soon as they wake up. Most smokers have their first cigarette with their first cup of coffee or after breakfast. A few smokers smoke in bed as soon as they wake up, even before brushing their teeth. Apparently, the intestinal systems of these smokers are accustomed to this ritual. No wonder they complain of constipation as soon as they give up smoking!

Over the years, coffee and cigarettes become stimulants for bowel movements. Your gastrointestinal system grows conditioned to the coffee-cigarette fix in the morning. Be prepared for some constipation for three to six days after giving up smoking, and consider using a mild stool softener (Metamucil, prune juice, among others) to regain regularity. If you smoke cigarettes as soon as you wake up, you will have a more difficult time parting with the habit than those who begin smoking later in the day. The longer the interval between waking up and having a cigarette, the easier it will be to give up the habit.

Also, the time interval that a smoker can sustain without smoking with minimum discomfort is very important. For example, if you can go four hours or more without a cigarette with minimal discomfort—at work, in movie theaters, on planes—you'll have a better chance of giving up the habit.

When You Smoke Your Last Cigarette of the Day

If you smoke the last cigarette of the day in bed or smoke during the night if your sleep is disturbed, expect to have a very hard time quitting, as the habit is firmly entrenched in your Instinctual Division. You tend to reach for a cigarette automatically. If you can reduce the number of cigarettes you smoke before quitting, you may have a somewhat easier time of it. At the very least, begin to pay attention to each cigarette, writing down the time and circumstances in your journal.

Your Smoking Triggers

Every smoker would agree that not all of the cigarettes they smoke give them pleasure. Over the years, the smoking habit slowly occupies the entire spectrum of their transactions with the world, so that on many occasions cigarettes are smoked for reasons other than deriving pleasure. Based on the information that many smokers have given me, I believe that a smoker has three basic triggers for smoking—instinctual, compelled, and intentional.

INSTINCTUAL SMOKING

Instinctual smoking is triggered by an activity or setting. For example, many of my patients report that they automatically light a cigarette when they pick up the phone. Most of the time they are not even consciously aware that they are doing it. Another instinctual setting is driving a car. No smoker has ever given me a satisfactory explanation for such a strong relationship between cigarettes and these activities. In my opinion, a telephone call represents an implied invasion of a smoker's privacy or a momentary disruption—even when it's a friendly call. This requires compensatory consolation through a mechanism smokers have come to trust. Similarly, driving alone is a boring task. To remain alert, awake, and occupied, smokers find that cigarettes come in very handy. Smoking can break the monotony of a long drive or a long wait.

Between 50 and 60 percent of a day's total cigarettes fall in the category of instinctual smoking. Smokers are conditioned to reach for a cigarette automatically when they are involved in such activities. A smoker can decrease the number of cigarettes smoked in this setup with little conscious effort. However, that's only half the battle.

If you are a strong instinctual smoker, it is important to understand that it will take four to five weeks after the last puff for instinctual triggers to fade or disappear from your mind. Knowing this will help you prepare realistically for the period after you take your last puff.

COMPELLED SMOKING

About 20 to 50 percent of cigarettes are smoked for an explicit, expressed need. Smokers come to rely on cigarettes to hone their performance. For example, people like artists, writers, and strategists use cigarettes to isolate themselves in their own world, to come up with creative ideas. Sensitive, fragile, and anxiety-prone smokers use cigarettes as tranquilizers, and they tend to do more compelled and less instinctual smoking than other smokers. Smokers with a sense of insecurity, an inferiority complex, and low self-esteem tend to insulate themselves from the world through this habit. Smokers are frightened of giving up compelled smoking, and if the percentage they smoke due to a compulsion is higher than 50 percent, this fear becomes a severe barrier.

Many smokers from this category smoke more cigarettes after they decide to stop smoking up until the moment they quit. If these individuals are relatively healthy, it is extremely difficult to convince them to give up compelled smoking. These smokers demand advanced assurances that they can survive without cigarettes before their last cigarette.

If you fall into this category, it is important to remind yourself that you must believe in yourself and your innate talents more than in cigarettes. By accomplishing this transformation, you not only become a comfortable nonsmoker but also a stress-free, confident, and delightful individual.

INTENTIONAL SMOKING

The remaining 10 to 20 percent of the total cigarettes consumed by the average smoker are intentionally used to derive pleasure. There are certain times in the day—in the early morning with coffee, at a lunch break, after dinner, after sex, or in a social setting, when most smokers enjoy their cigarettes to the maximum. In fact, this small fraction of intentional smoking becomes a major obstacle to a smoker in his struggle to stop smoking. After the last puff, the struggle index peaks during the period of intentional smoking, unleashing pangs of cravings for cigarettes. To ease this intense discomfort, smokers hunt for substitutes, such as candy, cookies, and rich foods. To gratify the need that used to be filled by intentional smoking, many smokers gain twenty to thirty pounds after giving up the smoking habit. Intentional smoking tempts a smoker to pick up a cigarette for weeks and months after the last puff.

The only way to resolve this situation is to fully accept that you must sacrifice the pleasure derived from smoking, thus neutralizing the Deprivation Drive. There is no other choice.

The Influence of Weight Issues

Smoking is an appetite suppressant, not because it contains nicotine but because it dulls the senses of taste and smell. Many people have learned to control their weight by smoking cigarettes. In fact, the mere mention of weight gain prevents many female smokers from even attempting to quit. If they do quit and gain weight, they more easily slide back into the habit. A smoker who is already obese or constantly struggles with weight will find it harder to give up smoking. This is a perception issue more than a health issue. It does not help to admonish a person that a ten-pound weight gain is a small price to pay for one's health.

If you have a weight problem and want to give up cigarettes, you are facing a formidable challenge. Giving up smoking may be a one-shot deal, but losing and maintaining a specific weight is an ongoing struggle. As it is, losing weight in the presence of abundant food is one of the toughest hurdles. On top of this challenge, your body is overloaded with the task of giving up smoking. It's best not to try doing too much all at once. If you are significantly overweight, my advice is to take control of your weight-loss program first. A strict diet-management program requires a lot of patience and rigor that can help you fight the smoking habit in the future. Once you are comfortable with your weight-management program, you can turn your attention to the smoking habit. If you have to lose only a very little weight, a minor adjustment will enable you to accomplish both at the same time.

If, however, you need to stop smoking due to health reasons, you may have no choice but to stop smoking first. The up side is that you will then be able to take advantage of the increased pulmonary reserve to exercise on a regular basis and attempt to lose weight later on. But the ideal approach is to lose weight first, then embark on giving up smoking at a later date.

Number of Attempts to Quit

Giving up smoking is not an easy task. One peculiar feature of this habit (indeed, of most habits) is that the first attempt to quit is the easiest, and that's when a smoker has the best chance of winning. Irrespective of the technique—cold turkey, hypnosis, acupuncture, the patch—the first attempt will be the most successful. Unfortunately, many people go back to smoking because they perceived it wasn't that hard to quit, and they're in for a big shock the next time they try.

If you're trying to quit for the second time, you have to understand two important facts:

1. Using the same method the second time around will have little or no effect, and you'll have to choose a different technique. For example, if acupuncture or the patch was helpful in curbing the urges the first time, it is useless for the second and subsequent attempts.
2. Even with the help of a better and more powerful technique, the urge to smoke will be a lot stronger

compared to that of your first attempt to quit. You have a tougher struggle to succeed the second time and thereafter. Having learned a valuable lesson from your failed attempts, you may have a tendency to stay off cigarettes in your subsequent attempts for the rest of your life. This certainly confirms that human beings appreciate the results only if they endure a certain amount of hardship.

The Influence of Other Habits

If cigarette smoking is your only counterproductive habit, you're in much better shape than those with other compulsions such as alcohol, drugs, or chemical dependencies.

Alcohol is definitely an obstacle in a smoker's path. After many years of their not smoking, I have seen people return to the habit when under the influence of alcohol. Over the years, alcohol and smoking establish an inseparable partnership, making it very difficult for smokers to give up cigarettes alone. But giving up alcohol and smoking simultaneously is extremely difficult. Many recovered alcoholics smoke with a vengeance once they stop drinking because they find comfort in cigarettes.

Smoking marijuana or using psychotropic drugs will impede the effort to stop smoking cigarettes. I usually urge my patients to give up these other habits before attempting to stop smoking.

Sometimes patients come to see me, wanting to give up only a single habit even though they are hooked on more than one. These patients pick the habit they consider more important to rid from their lives. As a professional, it is my job to understand the whole picture and present it to my patients. Let's take a close look at a few situations to understand when smoking cessation can be a priority and when it may not be.

SITUATION 1: IT'S HARD TO BREAK ALCOHOL AND SMOKING ADDICTIONS SIMULTANEOUSLY

A person with a history of pulmonary lung disease and mild heart problems wants to quit smoking. But he is also a heavy alcohol consumer. In this case, it's important to understand that unconsciously people demand some kind of compensation for giving up an attractive, pleasure-producing addictive habit. Even though it is a voluntary attempt on their part to give up their habit, they still look for a substitute to fill the void. Alcohol is a handy surrogate, but one that will almost certainly sabotage success. When people try to quit smoking first, with the intention of tackling a drinking habit later, they almost always go back to smoking. Alcohol is a mind-altering addictive drug, and it prevents people from keeping their guard up. Vigilance goes down the drain, and the next thing they know, they're smoking again.

On those rare occasions that an individual must stop smoking immediately for health reasons, I convince the person to stop drinking for a few weeks after the last puff. But I also insist that he should tone down his alcohol consumption for the remainder of his life. I warn my patient that the threat of picking up a cigarette is always alive and definitely more so in the presence of alcohol. By not allowing a person to drink alcohol on a temporary basis, I am overcoming my patient's objections to quitting drinking as well as decreasing the potential of failure during the initial stage of his fight. After eight to twelve weeks, he will settle down to a new smoke-free lifestyle and may not look toward alcohol as a substitute.

SITUATION 2: ALCOHOLISM RECOVERY
PRESENTS A CHALLENGE TO SMOKERS

A patient used to be an alcoholic and a cigarette smoker. He has managed to give up drinking but is now seeking my help in giving up smoking. The rule of thumb is that it is always difficult to give up the last habit, because when people give up the first habit, inadvertently they fall back on the second habit as a crutch. Unfortunately, when they attempt to give up their last habit, they have nothing to hang on to. I have come across patients who were dry for more than ten years, but they still had to struggle harder than other smokers to give up smoking. Having said that, it is clear to me that recovering alcoholics also have a gift when it comes to breaking the last habit. They have already geared themselves for battle. They crave freedom from the slavery of addiction and have already proved to themselves that they can overcome the emotional barriers.

SITUATION 3: GIVING UP
MARIJUANA AND CIGARETTES

If an individual is in the habit of smoking both marijuana and cigarettes, and is attempting to give up smoking only marijuana but not cigarettes, he can do so without fail. The pleasure derived from smoking marijuana is not from the smoke itself, as in the case of cigarettes, but is due to the absorption of an active chemical agent (tetrahydrocannabinol) by the lungs, which is released into the bloodstream and carried to the brain. Thus, smoking cigarettes does not trigger a strong desire to smoke marijuana.

But attempting to give up cigarettes without giving up marijuana is rarely possible for two reasons. The first reason is that marijuana is a mind-altering drug. Even intermittent usage of mind-altering drugs or alcohol can make it difficult to regain full control over smoking. The second reason is that smoking marijuana physically resembles smoking cigarettes, thereby triggering the desire to smoke cigarettes.

BREAKING THE HABIT: JUST SAY NO

Several years ago, Roger, a forty-four-year-old advertising director, came to see me to give up the cigarette smoking habit. During the interview, Roger told me that he smoked three or four joints of marijuana a week, and he was not willing to give up that pleasure. Despite my advice to discontinue both habits at the same time, he stuck to his guns and chose to give up only cigarettes. At first, Roger was successful, and he remained cigarette-free for several months. He reported to me in a pleased voice that he had been able to continue smoking marijuana without its triggering any desire for a cigarette. As far as he was concerned, the two habits were completely separate entities. Then, a year after he quit smoking cigarettes, Roger lost his job in a company layoff. He began to smoke more marijuana—two joints a day—in an effort to relieve his stress. In a weak moment, he bummed a cigarette at a party.

When Roger returned to my office, three years after his first visit, he was back to smoking both cigarettes and marijuana. "This time I'm serious about quitting both habits," he said humbly. Roger understood what I had been trying to tell him. Now, five years later, he is still free from both habits.

The Influence of Prescription Drugs

If an individual takes prescription medications to treat attention deficit disorder (ADD or ADHD), anxiety, neurosis, or depression, he can expect to have a very hard time quitting his smoking habit.

Your Frame of Mind

Don't underestimate the importance of timing. The timing of your attack on the smoking habit is extremely important. In life, timing is the essence of a winning strategy. A perfect example is the Allied invasion of Normandy—the final, all-out attack against Hitler and his forces. The Allied leaders invested their entire hope of winning the war on this crucial move. The field commanders were setting up the stage, whereas the commanding generals focused on picking the perfect time for the invasion. History has revealed that the combination of precise timing and perfect execution by the western military alliances literally changed the tide of this war. The invasion of Normandy was the beginning of the end of Hitler's barbaric, brutal regime.

Likewise, the timing of your attack on the smoking habit calls for careful consideration. The popular concept among behavioral therapists is that no time is better than the present to take action against an addictive habit. In theory, it sounds right. But the cold light of reality presents a different picture. I am convinced that there is a tremendous advantage in a well-prepared, preemptive attack against the smoking habit.

You need to look around you and realistically evaluate your

circumstances. For example, if you are in the middle of a messy divorce proceeding, it is highly unlikely that you can totally ignore your personal problems and concentrate on ending your smoking habit. To quit smoking is to wage battle with an enemy within, and it is easy for this enemy to understand your state of mind and sabotage your efforts. Do not expect any sympathy or understanding from your archenemy. Every failed attempt will further erode your confidence and strengthen the enemy's hand.

When you are in a state of depression or distress, the primitive emotions demand adequate compensation by associating with a pleasure-seeking device. The threat of losing a job or a sickness in the family can rattle you and affect your composure. We all know this from experience, and it is foolish to ignore reality. It is likely that, feeling depressed and despondent, you will seek refuge in your old comfort, instead of fighting the habit.

Your chances of success will be greater if your life is in balance when you take on the task of quitting smoking. That is the ideal scenario. However, life does not always cooperate by presenting the perfect timing. That's why my method includes exercises to reinforce your spirits as you confront your enemy.

Your Depth-of-Addiction Score

Refined, disciplined, and dignified human behavior is like a well-maintained, manicured garden where a handpicked collection of color-coordinated shrubs, floral plants, hedges, and trees grace the landscape. This dream garden is the result of pride, good imagination, and dedicated hard work. The same holds true for refined behavior. Addictive habits are the untended weeds and crabgrass in the garden of our behavior complex. The longer the duration of our neglect, the harder it is to restore our behavior to acceptable standards. Recognizing the presence of a destructive, addictive habit in a person's life is the beginning of the end of that habit. And taming such a habit is the final frontier in the saga of an addictive habit.

The following Depth of Addiction Score will help you evaluate your personal level of attachment to your habit. The stronger your attachment, the greater your difficulty in quitting.

The Depth-of-Addiction Meter

Circle the number in each category that applies to your habit.

AGE YOU STARTED SMOKING	Under 18	3
	18–25	1
	Over 25	0
TYPE OF CIGARETTE SMOKED	Menthol	1
	Nonmenthol	0
NUMBER OF CIGARETTES DAILY	More than 2 packs	3
	2 packs or less	2
WHEN YOU SMOKE YOUR FIRST CIGARETTE OF THE DAY	Within 20 minutes of rising	3
	Within 2 hours of rising	2
	Later in the day	1
WHEN YOU SMOKE YOUR LAST CIGARETTE OF THE DAY	In bed before you go to sleep	3
	In the middle of the night if you wake up	2
	At least an hour before bedtime	1

SMOKING TRIGGERS	Higher percentage of intentional smoking	3
	Higher percentage of compelled smoking	2
	Higher percentage of instinctual smoking	1
SMOKING AND WEIGHT ISSUES	Obese or constantly struggling with weight	3
	Normal weight but worried about gaining	2
	Normal weight but not worried about gaining	0
PREVIOUS ATTEMPTS TO QUIT	More than 3 serious attempts	3
	1–3 serious attempts	2
	Never tried to quit	0
INFLUENCE OF OTHER HABITS (circle all that apply)	Often smoke while drinking alcohol	3
	Also smoke marijuana	3
	Take psychotropic medications	2
	Take anti-anxiety prescription medications	1
STRESS LEVEL	Extremely distressed over events or circumstances	3
	Mildly stressed	2
	Relatively comfortable	1

Total: Add up the circled numbers. This is your total score. Enter it here and in the Smoking Cessation Struggle Index calculator on page 111.

Now that you have a clear picture of your habit and the power it exerts over you, you have taken the first step in reasserting control over your life. Now let's examine your underlying motivations for smoking—those invisible drives that form the emotional basis of your Addictive Profile.

Identify Your Addictive Profile

TO BE EFFECTIVE against the smoking habit, you must focus on the invisible enemy—the internally generated drives that feed it. By fixating on the external features, you may stop picking up a cigarette but you will never get rid of the compulsion or the desire to smoke. As long as the compulsion is alive, you will eventually return to the habit. You cannot break a habit by getting rid of the offending substance.

The key to beating the addictive habit is the underlying drives that comprise your Addictive Profile. These drives are always lurking in the background of the habit. The stress of these drives primes the craving to smoke. Think of the mind of a smoker as an emotional pressure cooker, fed by one or more elements of the Addictive Profile. As the pressure builds, the smoker experiences a growing discomfort, exhibited by agitation, rage, sleeplessness, the inability to concentrate, and so on. Most of my patients say they feel a battle going on in their mind, a void in the pit of their stomach, and an all-encompassing sadness. The longer the hardened smoker stays away from cigarettes, the more preoccupied his mind becomes. The stress builds. At some point, when the psychological pressure becomes unbearable, the desire to smoke turns into a ravaging craving to release the pressure.

These intense cravings are not, as many people believe, caused by nicotine withdrawal. They're caused by an emotional need. That need comes from deeply rooted stories about why smoking is beneficial or necessary. The emotional drive of these stories allows people to continue behaviors that the rational mind clearly acknowledges as destructive. These drives are all-consuming. Often a person will have more than one of them. They trigger the Emotional Division to seek relief.

Many professionals in the field of addiction believe that, for an addict, the urge to smoke cigarettes or to consume alcohol or drugs is mainly physical, not psychological. I totally reject this concept. An individual is driven mentally to enjoy the attractive, beneficial experience from the addictive habit. The overwhelming urge an addict feels to pursue the habit is strictly mental, not physical. The physical release from the addiction happens relatively quickly, once the toxins are flushed from the body. But the nucleus remains—the overwhelming sense of deprivation, entitlement, invincibility, disenchantment, insecurity, and defiance that gave rise to the addiction in the first place.

None of us is completely free of these drives. They are integral to human emotions, and in a proper balance can even enhance our lives and motivate us to achieve. However, for an addict, one or more of these drives take on a pathological character. For example, the normal influence of the Insecurity Drive is necessary to keep you alert and vigilant, thus enabling your survival. An overactive Insecurity Drive paralyzes you and impairs your ability to make decisions. It also fosters dependency by encouraging you to rely on an external crutch to get you through the day.

The Addictive Profile, which is formed by an imbalance in one or more of these drives, is the engine that charges up addictive behavior. In this section, we will examine the drives of the Addictive Profile more closely, showing how an imbalance of one or more drives helps to keep you addicted. Take the quiz that is provided for each drive to determine whether it is out of balance for you. The results of these quizzes will provide essential clues to the nature of your addiction.

The Deprivation Drive

A healthy fear of deprivation can be a positive motivator. It's what gets you up in the morning and sends you off to work to provide for yourself and your family. Being without food and shelter is true deprivation. No one needs cigarettes to survive, but you'd have a hard time convincing the smoker whose habit is compelled by the Deprivation Drive of this fact. The smoker fears deprivation—that moment of emptiness when the person used to reach for a cigarette and it is no longer there. Most of the current treatments to help smokers quit focus on filling up that emptiness. They don't look at the individual—the smoker—and ask why this person is addicted to puffing sticks of tobacco. Instead, they try to pacify the fear. They give the smoker doses of nicotine through patches and pills, inhalers, and plastic "cigarettes" that allow the person to mimic the action of smoking. They use antidepressants to ease the tension of giving up the habit. None of these substitutes works for long, because the smoker still has the need to be pacified. The feeling of deprivation remains.

For example, my patient Samantha started smoking when she was in college. She found that smoking helped her concentrate on her homework and kept her awake during long nights of study. The relationship continued when she became a successful trial attorney. The night before a trial, Samantha burned the midnight oil and smoked feverishly. She resisted giving up cigarettes for years because she feared losing her dynamic character and forceful handling of cases. Her confidence rested on an alliance with her smoking habit. Samantha's first question to me was, "Will I be as effective after I quit smoking?"

When Samantha visualized her smoking habit, she saw an empty place inside herself that was instantly filled when she inhaled the warm smoke from her cigarette. Every time she imagined herself at her desk, working furiously, she thought about what it would be like to reach out and find nothing there. Her chest clutched in anticipation of the deprivation. She had equated energy with that thin stick of tobacco for so long that she didn't know how to separate herself from her habit. Only when she finally grasped the fact that there was no real deprivation, no real energy drain, except as an idea in her mind, could she overcome her fear.

Is your Deprivation Drive out of balance? Take the following quiz to determine whether it plays a significant role in your smoking habit.

QUIZ: YOUR DEPRIVATION QUOTIENT

Read the following statements. In the box, give yourself
1 point for each statement that you agree with,
and 0 if it doesn't describe you.

STATEMENT	VALUE
You often feel physically tired or "burned out," especially toward the end of the day.	
You feel as if others are better off than you.	
You are easily bored.	
You often wish you had more friends.	
You have problems forming lasting relationships.	
You are easily overwhelmed by ordinary challenges, such as a broken pipe, a failed recipe, or a traffic jam.	
You think others have more opportunities or are luckier than you.	
You dislike your job, or the treatment you receive from your boss or colleagues.	
You wish you had a spouse who could better understand your needs.	
You have a low tolerance for emotional discomfort.	

Score: Total the numbers in the right-hand column. That is your deprivation
quotient. If your score is 1–5, you have a relatively normal Deprivation Drive.
If your score is more than 5, your Deprivation Drive is overactive, making it
a factor in your smoking habit.

The Entitlement Drive

A balanced sense of entitlement is important to your self-esteem. It allows you to feel special and motivates you to take care of yourself because your life is worth something. However, entitlement does not exist in the physical world. Nature does not play favorites. It does not give you a break because you work hard, or you're a nice person, or you're a genius. It does not care about your problems. Its terms and conditions are clear: behaviors have consequences. Just because you think you're entitled to reduce stress with a cigarette doesn't mean you'll avoid the many dire consequences associated with the habit. If your Entitlement Drive is overactive, you ignore nature's rules.

Recently, I worked with a patient named Mark, an executive with a large financial company, who came to me to help him overcome his smoking habit. Mark explained to me in our first session that he had tried and failed many times to give up smoking. This was a man accustomed to winning. He was embarrassed by his failure.

When I asked him why he smoked, he explained to me that he worked long hours every day in a very stressful environment. Smoking helped to relax him; it eased the stress somewhat. "I need that relief," he said.

What he was really saying was, "I deserve to seek comfort from chemicals and not pay the price." But every bad habit has a price.

In this day and age, I see how we have pampered ourselves. We want what we want when we want it. And when we don't get what we feel are our just desserts—even if it is only a moment of comfort from a cigarette or a couple of glasses of wine at the end of the day—we are angry and resentful, as if we are being robbed.

I asked Mark, "Do you think you get a pass because you are good, or hardworking, or smart?" He laughed at the idea. He could see it was foolish. Before we could begin to tackle the problem of Mark's addiction, we first had to establish the lie he was telling himself. We had to reacquaint him with the world as it was, not as he wished it to be.

There is great power in acknowledging your place in the world, but many people cannot see this because they are obsessed with what others think and are only interested in imitating others since it feels good. Their reasoning is, "Other people feel entitled to a reward for their efforts, so why shouldn't I have one, too?" Unfortunately, it is folly to follow the trend set by others without acknowledging the price tag of the reward.

Is your Entitlement Drive out of balance? Take the following quiz to determine whether it plays a significant role in your smoking habit.

QUIZ: YOUR ENTITLEMENT QUOTIENT

Read the following statements. In the box, give yourself
1 point for each statement that you agree with,
and 0 if it doesn't describe you.

STATEMENT	VALUE
You often think that you work harder than those around you, and if something is going to get done, you have to do it yourself.	

You feel entitled to kick back and take a break every so often.	
You think you're justified in not always following the rules.	
You often feel that others do not understand you.	
You believe that hard work and accomplishment should be rewarded in a tangible way.	
You tend to seek instant gratification.	
You consider yourself special.	
When you see something you want, you buy it.	
You smoke in the house and the car, even though your smoking bothers family members.	
You often feel as if you deserve more.	

Score: Total the numbers in the right-hand column. That is your entitlement quotient. If your score is 1–5, you have a relatively normal Entitlement Drive. If your score is more than 5, your Entitlement Drive is overactive, making it a factor in your smoking habit.

The Invincibility Drive

No human being is invincible, but this drive can have a limited positive effect. It's the underlying sense of personal power that gives us courage in seemingly impossible situations. Out of balance, however, the Invincibility Drive is pure arrogance. It will stop you dead in your tracks. You are not God. You are not omnipotent. The smoker with an Invincibility Drive doesn't really think smoking will harm him. He believes that smoking only hurts others. He believes that he is strong enough to withstand the wrath of his addiction. He is special.

Neil, a forty-one-year-old police captain, came to see me to stop smoking. He had been trying to give up smoking for about four years without success. Once, with great difficulty, he had managed to stop for three days, using willpower. During that time he could not concentrate on any of his activities and he told me he was enormously agitated. Finally, the strain of not smoking was too great and he caved in.

Neil told me that quitting aids, like the patch and nicotine gum, didn't even make a dent in his habit. This puzzled him. "Doctor, I can do anything if I put my mind to it. How come I can't do this?"

"Let's figure it out," I said. I asked him a few questions and slowly began to see how Neil had succumbed to the Invincibility Drive.

A handsome, muscular six-footer, Neil oozed confidence and ambition. In high school he'd played football and tennis and excelled at both. He was also academically successful, with excellent grades that earned him placement at a prestigious university. He majored in languages and graduated with honors. At the time he came to my office, Neil was close to earning his law degree, and he aspired to become a district attorney or a judge.

I felt that Neil was somewhat cocky and slightly overconfident about his abilities. He had started to smoke in college; he liked smoking and found that it helped him to concentrate on his studies without getting bored. He smoked just under a pack a day and said he enjoyed most of the cigarettes. He admitted that he didn't think smoking would really hurt him.

"Why are you so anxious to stop if you don't think cigarettes are harming you?" I asked.

"It's an image thing," he replied. "Smokers are social pariahs. People look down on you. I find that intolerable."

With a guy like Neil, I knew I would have to fight fire with fire. I had to shake up his pride and sense of invincibility. "You see yourself as a very capable, strong guy," I said. "But here's the truth. The minute you decided to stop smoking and failed to do so, you became a slave to your habit. There is no two ways about it. Whether smoking is harmful or not is immaterial. When push comes to shove, you could not conquer your weakness. I wonder how you expect to change the world around you if you cannot change this one thing in your own life."

Neil recoiled from my harsh words as if struck. They stung. But after a few minutes' reflecting on what I had told him, he said firmly, "I will stop smoking." As he left my office, he said, "I guess it's time for me to take a good dose of humility."

I didn't hear from Neil again for several weeks. Finally he called and said, "I have been a nonsmoker for three weeks, Doc. I'm on my way to being a comfortable nonsmoker."

Is your Invincibility Drive out of balance? Take the following quiz to determine whether it plays a significant role in your smoking habit.

QUIZ: YOUR INVINCIBILITY QUOTIENT

Read the following statements. In the box, give yourself
1 point for each statement that you agree with,
and 0 if it doesn't describe you.

STATEMENT	VALUE
So far, you've experienced no real health problems from smoking.	
You like to cite exceptions to the rule, such as smokers who live to be 100.	
You think of yourself as exceptionally strong.	
You like to beat the odds—in sports and at work.	
You are not impressed with authority.	
You march to your own drummer.	
You believe smoking gives you a performance edge.	
You are highly successful in your profession.	
You like to take risks, and engage in activities such as gambling or skydiving or bungee jumping.	
You have no patience for stupidity.	

Score: Total the numbers in the right-hand column. That is your invincibility quotient. If your score is 1–5, you have a relatively normal Invincibility Drive. If your score is more than 5, your Invincibility Drive is overactive, making it a factor in your smoking habit.

The Disenchantment Drive

Disenchantment is a necessary part of being human. We all have disappointments in life, and if we keep them in perspective, we can learn from them. Our of balance, however, disenchantment can spiral into a sense of overwhelming gloom—the feeling that life has robbed you of joy. The wider the disparity between your expectations and actual reality, the deeper the disenchantment. Many people who are diagnosed as clinically depressed are actually experiencing disenchantment. The Disenchantment Drive can play a role in smoking addiction when depression triggers a heavy reliance on a crutch just to see you through the day. Smokers compelled by disenchantment are less likely to worry about the consequences.

Paul came to see me to stop smoking, and in the course of our consultation he also admitted that he had a marijuana habit, smoking three or four joints a day. At twenty-eight, he had achieved tremendous success as a screenwriter. He had the magic touch, and his films were big hits. He was definitely born with a talent to stretch his imagination and produce tales of adventure, intrigue, and romance. However, Paul was also a shy, sensitive, and sentimental man, who hated what he perceived as the manipulative and diabolical world of Hollywood. Over the years he had learned to deal with the harsh environment around him by retreating into the fantasies of his creation. In these fantasies he could have absolute control over the sequence of events and their outcome. Not so in his life. In the real world, nature and the actions of others control most events, and you cannot predict the outcome. Individuals have limitations in their ability to shape life to their liking.

Paul could not stand the ugliness of his Hollywood environment, which was so different from his gentle, romantic fantasies about the way things should be. He was disenchanted. Smoking cigarettes and marijuana helped him cope, but his habits had begun to take a toll on his health, spirits, and relationship with his beautiful actress wife. Lately, he had begun to notice that marijuana was undermining his creative abilities. When he came to see me, he was frightened. He said, "I'm damned if I stop, and I'm damned if I don't."

I told Paul there was a way out for him. He did not have to live the rest of his life overwhelmed by a Disenchantment Drive. He could learn to bring his expectations into line with reality and become a sensible, sensitive, good-natured pragmatist. He could have the best of both worlds.

Is your Disenchantment Drive out of balance? Take the following quiz to determine whether it plays a significant role in your smoking habit.

QUIZ: YOUR DISENCHANTMENT QUOTIENT

Read the following statements. In the box, give yourself 1 point for each statement that you agree with, and 0 if it doesn't describe you.

STATEMENT	VALUE
You have not had the life you dreamed of.	
You consider yourself a romantic.	

You think others succeed because they have inside connections or special advantages.	
You spend a lot of time in solitary pursuits.	
You have been sexually molested by someone you know.	
You often drink to excess or use recreational drugs to give you an edge and help you feel good.	
You are highly creative but have trouble executing your ideas.	
You tend to have a fatalistic attitude about smoking—what will be will be.	
You have been treated for depression.	
You often feel bored.	

Score: Total the numbers in the right-hand column. That is your disenchantment quotient. If your score is 1–5, you have a relatively normal Disenchantment Drive. If your score is more than 5, your Disenchantment Drive is overactive, making it a factor in your smoking habit.

The Insecurity Drive

The Insecurity Drive is the opposite of the Invincibility Drive. In proper balance these two drives give you a realistic idea of your potential. Out of balance, the Insecurity Drive involves a lack of courage to face the uncertain future and a lack of confidence in one's ability to tackle the challenges of a harsh world. Individuals with this drive hesitate to take action because they cannot be assured of the result. They forget that no human being has certainty about the future. They expect absolute reassurance that everything will work out fine. In the absence of this, they fret endlessly over minor issues. They are not proactive; they only know how to react. They long for peace of mind, but they never find it. Instead, they end up agitated, anxious, and sleep deprived.

In this quest to seek relief from their plight, they turn to substances that will numb their anxieties. We've all witnessed individuals who smoke like chimneys, binge on food, or gulp down alcohol, saying they do it to calm their nerves. Yet they are the most nervous people we know!

Janice was a thirty-year-old woman who had been seeing a psychiatrist for several years to treat her social anxiety disorder. She told me that she had always been shy, but her shyness had grown into an extreme aversion to any kind of socializing. She would have a panic attack at the very idea of going to a party or meeting friends for dinner. The psychiatrist prescribed the anti-anxiety drug Ativan, but it did little to ease her tension. Janice smoked three packs of cigarettes a day, often lighting one as soon as the last had been extinguished. By the time she came to me, she was addicted to both Ativan and cigarettes, and neither had relieved her social anxiety. If anything, she was even more reclusive than she had been before.

I asked Janice to tell me about herself. She explained that she had suffered from low self-esteem and feelings of inadequacy since she was a child. Her mother was a great beauty, who had once been a professional fashion model. "But as you can see,

Doctor, I am no great beauty. I take after my father, not my mother."

All her life, Janice felt she had stood in her mother's shadow. She had few friends, men weren't interested in her, and she was trying to come to terms with being alone in life, because she would never be attractive. However, she said, it was very hard to accept this reality without support from her habits, and she desperately wanted my help.

"I have news for you," I told Janice. "Your problem is not cigarettes or Ativan. It is insecurity based on your vanity. You feel betrayed because nature has not given you your mother's beauty. Therefore, you feel shortchanged. Besides your own insecurity, you are also angry at nature."

Janice's unhappiness about her physical appearance filled her with anxiety and self-consciousness in public settings. Eventually, she became bitter, depressed, and isolated. In effect, she became what she feared—socially awkward, professionally inadequate, sexually inhibited, and spiritually deprived. She turned to Ativan and smoking to loosen her up and relieve her anxieties, but these antidotes failed to solve her greatest problem— the passionate desire to be someone else.

Another of my patients, Serena, a forty-five-year-old, happily married woman, smoked less than a pack a day. For the most part, she could take them or leave them, except for the three or four cigarettes she smoked each night before bed. Whenever she tried to give up those cigarettes, she felt extremely agitated and could not sleep.

When Serena was thirteen, she lost her father, whom she loved very much. She remembered that her father always tucked her into bed with a cigarette in his hand while he narrated a short story. She felt calm and protected. A couple of years after her father's death, Serena picked up the smoking habit, probably as a sensory connection to her father. Later on in life, whenever she was scared, nervous, or upset, one puff was enough to calm her. I believed that Serena's nighttime cigarettes were a way of having her father tuck her into bed.

When I presented this simple thesis to Serena, her eyes grew wide with understanding. I could almost see the light click on in her mind. "Dr. Prasad," she said, "I never made that connection before. Now I know I can stop my habit."

Is your Insecurity Drive out of balance? Take the following quiz to determine whether it plays a significant role in your smoking habit.

QUIZ: YOUR INSECURITY QUOTIENT

Read the following statements. In the box, give yourself 1 point for each statement that you agree with, and 0 if it doesn't describe you.

STATEMENT	VALUE
You experience disturbed sleep.	
You are nervous and filled with anxiety in social settings.	
You worry that others watch you and judge you lacking.	
You are terrified of making a mistake.	

You consider yourself less attractive and less stylish than others.	
You grew up in an environment where adults were overly critical of you.	
You often feel lonely.	
You have trouble forming lasting relationships.	
If a friend cancels a date or your spouse is in a bad mood, you tend to assume you did something wrong.	
You don't believe you have the strength to stop smoking.	

Score: Total the numbers in the right-hand column. That is your insecurity quotient. If your score is 1–5, you have a relatively normal Insecurity Drive. If your score is more than 5, your Insecurity Drive is overactive, making it a factor in your smoking habit.

The Defiance Drive

We all need a little defiance in our lives. It's what distinguishes us from robots. However, defiance for its own sake can get us into trouble. Many times a smoker hangs on to the habit as a gesture of defiance. The zeal of this drive is such that the smoker doesn't even worry about the consequences of his behavior or his own quality of life. He consistently downplays the risks or outright ignores them. In most cases the Defiance Drive is fueled by the Invincibility Drive.

The rebellious tendency is more pronounced among adolescents, but it is usually softened as a person matures. Young rebels are likely to take up unproductive behaviors like smoking, recreational drug use, and alcohol use, and as they grow and become less adventurous, they may still retain traces of habits they acquired at an earlier age. In some cases, a person will become addicted to a habit that holds on long after the rebellious urge has passed. In other cases, the rebellion is so deep that a person holds on to the habit, refusing to yield, in the belief that it represents the very core of his identity.

Robert, a fifty-two-year-old oncologist, was the last person you'd ever expect to be a smoker. Tall and good-looking, he exuded the self-confidence typical of a doctor who battles medicine's deadliest foe. He was a relentless fighter when the lives of his patients were at stake, but he couldn't conquer his habit. Although Robert treated many people whose bodies were ravaged by the lifelong effects of cigarettes, and he knew that more than 90 percent of all lung cancers were directly attributable to smoking, he continued to smoke two packs of cigarettes a day.

Robert became a steady smoker when he was eleven, as an act of rebellion against his strict father. The incident that precipitated his habit was the time his father caught him smoking with friends and publicly berated and humiliated him. His smoking became an act of defiance. The fact that he continued forty-one years later was deeply frustrating to him, especially since the consequences were so great. He admitted to me that his habit had a negative impact on every area of his life. It compromised his credibility as a doctor, embarrassed him in front of his colleagues, and created friction in his marriage. It was also beginning to cause health problems. He was often short of breath. He suffered from a persistent cough, and he had high blood pressure.

As an oncologist, Robert certainly knew intellectually that smoking was bad. But deep down in his heart he believed that giving up smoking was tantamount to caving in to his father who had caused him to lose face in front of his friends so long ago. Smoking became a symbol of his Defiance Drive, but he was completely unaware of it. When I gave him my thoughts on the matter, he at first gaped in disbelief, then started laughing. He now felt he could address his habit with a clear mind.

Is your Defiance Drive out of balance? Take the following quiz to determine whether it plays a significant role in your smoking habit.

QUIZ: YOUR DEFIANCE QUOTIENT

Read the following statements. In the box, give yourself 1 point for each statement that you agree with, and 0 if it doesn't describe you.

STATEMENT	VALUE
You have a short temper.	
You believe you were born to change the world for the better, and you believe you can.	
Other people don't understand your good motives.	
You think you understand the true issues concerning humans better than most people.	

STATEMENT	VALUE
Many people you come across are hypocrites.	
Powerful people don't care about the little guy.	
You love to lead others but hate to follow.	
You believe that sometimes the end justifies the means.	
You've always had a troubled relationship with your parents.	
You believe you are a true individual.	

Score: Total the numbers in the right-hand column. That is your defiance quotient. If your score is 1–5, you have a relatively normal Defiance Drive. If your score is more than 5, your Defiance Drive is overactive, making it a factor in your smoking habit.

Your Addictive Profile Score

Review your scores for each of the six drives, and make a note of where your score is more than 5. If you have an imbalance in one drive, your total score is 1; two drives, 2; three drives, 3; and so on. Write the number below and on the following page in the Smoking Cessation Struggle Index.

Total Addictive Profile Score: _____

STEP 4

Make the Break

YOU'VE DONE YOUR RESEARCH, and you're now armed with a clear picture of who you are as a smoker. Now it's time to use that information to establish a new identity as a comfortable nonsmoker.

Calculate Your Smoking Cessation Struggle Index

Your scores in the previous sections will help you determine the difficulty of quitting and the potential pitfalls you face.

Write down your scores from the calculators in the previous section:

1. Reasons for quitting _____.
2. Depth-of-Addiction meter _____.
3. Addictive Profile _____

Add the three numbers. This is your total score. Refer to the table below to determine how long you can expect to spend in each cessation grade.

Your Discomfort Score					
SCORE	GRADE 4	GRADE 3	GRADE 2	GRADE 1	TOTAL QUITTING TIME
40 or over	2 weeks	6 weeks	12 weeks	32 weeks	**52 weeks**
30–39	10 days	4 weeks	10 weeks	24 weeks	**40 weeks**
20–29	1 week	3 weeks	8 weeks	20 weeks	**32 weeks**
14–19	4 days	2 weeks	4 weeks	16 weeks	**23 weeks**
Less than 14	2 days	10 days	3 weeks	12 weeks	**17 weeks**

The clock starts ticking after the last puff. If you have even one puff, the clock will stop and restart from the beginning. It is extremely difficult to survive grade 4 discomfort for more than a week. Strive to shorten the period of grade 4 discomfort so you can move to a lower, more doable, grade.

Taking Your Last Puff

There are two ways to arrive at the last puff. The first method is to gradually increase the time interval between cigarettes and taper the consumption down to zero. With this method, initially you may find it easy to slash the number of cigarettes. But as you come closer to the last puff, you'll have to work harder to resist the temptation of smoking, and that can be exhausting. In the end, you may be left with very little energy to take the big leap from the last puff to no puff. Normally, I don't recommend a gradual approach. However, some people with scores of 40 or more find they need to make some inroads to reduce their scores before quitting altogether.

The best way to quit is to pick a time and place to terminate the habit in one shot. This method enables you to pool all your strength to inflict a mortal blow on your enemy in a single stroke. Make a serious ritual of it, even writing a contract to yourself to reinforce your commitment. State that commitment in irrevocable terms. People will often say, "I'm going to try to quit smoking." This is not a commitment, only a wish. Would you tell a landlord, "I'm going to try to pay the rent every month?" Would you tell your employer, "I'm going to try to get to the office on time every day?" Of course not. You'd soon be out of an apartment and a job. I urge you to bring the same level of commitment to the task of quitting your habit as you do to other important areas of your life. Think of it as a contract you are making with yourself that has no escape clause. To be successful, the contract must include:

- A decision to tackle the habit on its terms and conditions, not those you imagine or invent
- A decision that failure is not an option
- A decision to be not just free of the habit but *comfortable* and *productive* without the habit
- A decision that you, not your habit, will decide your fate

The Four Stages of Quitting

The course you will endure after the last puff is related to your ranking. Remember, the physical separation from cigarettes alone is not going to pave the path for a trouble-free, comfortable, nonsmoking lifestyle. The psychological adjustment to a nonsmoker's lifestyle is a time-consuming, grueling, and steady acclimatization process. You will pass through four critical stages to transform yourself from an uncomfortable smoker to a comfortable nonsmoker. Each stage is governed by a specific time frame and bound by precise withdrawal symptoms. However, your ability to go smoothly from stage to stage is in large part contingent on your level of discomfort.

Your Addictive Profile will play a role in this process. I have found that different drives tend to assert themselves more vigorously at various stages, and these impediments are detailed below.

STAGE 1: LAST PUFF TO ONE WEEK

Stage 1 of the quitting process is triggered after the last puff. Usually this stage extends up to one week. You will be besieged by pangs of strong urges to smoke, lasting for two to three minutes at least once every hour. You may feel that you have very little time to recover from the previous attack before the next urge surfaces. Preoccupation with smoking makes it difficult for you to concentrate on your daily tasks. You may experience dizzy spells and a sense of imbalance. You may constantly take deep breaths to fill the emptiness in your lungs and drink lots of water to wash off the peculiar taste in your mouth. Your hands will feel restless—you won't know what to do with them. Your sleep pattern will be disturbed, and you will feel exhausted at the end of the day.

Most people blame the depleting blood nicotine level for the discomfort experienced during this stage. This statement is partially true. Many smokers have said that they get about a 10 to 15 percent level of relief from nicotine-replacement supplements. But after two or three days, a smoker is tempted to have one deep drag from his favorite brand to extinguish the fire of deprivation once and for all. Unfortunately, one puff is enough to offset the advantage gained in this battle and puts him back at the very beginning of this stage. With each puff, the smoker extends the misery beyond another seven days. No one can withstand this stage for more than one week. The strategy of a smoker is to keep this stage as short and as comfortable as possible. Remember, the lower your scores, the shorter the duration of the first stage.

Factor in Your Addictive Profile

During Stage 1, the Deprivation Drive and the Insecurity Drive are the most prominent, so you need to be vigilant if your scores for these drives showed an imbalance.

The Deprivation Drive will provoke an insatiable desire to fill the void left behind by the smoking habit. Anticipate feelings of deprivation, and address them by taking long, slow deep breaths when you feel the urge to smoke or by brushing your teeth or drinking a glass of water with lemon. Try to avoid junk food during this stage. What appears at first to be a fair and innocent trade-off (food for cigarettes) may leave you in disarray. Many smokers turn back to smoking because of unacceptable weight gain. If you can hang in tight for at least seven days, it is possible to jump over the hump and enter into the second stage.

The Insecurity Drive will plant seeds of doubt that you can succeed, especially if you've tried to quit before but failed. You may be helped by being part of a group of smokers determined to quit. Seeing that others are in the same boat and having supportive company in your endeavor can build your courage.

STAGE 2: FROM FOUR TO SIX WEEKS

The second stage lasts from four to six weeks. You may experience short spells of a strong desire to smoke, lasting from two to three minutes once every three to four hours. You'll also experience a weak desire to smoke several times, spaced between strong urges. You'll tend to seek substitutions, such as munching on snacks or sweets to overcome your urges. You'll have to work harder to withstand this level of discomfort. The hallmark of the second stage is the loosening of the tight steel grip of the habit. You'll begin to feel a slight sense of confidence. By the midpoint of this stage, a glimmer of hope will surface. For the first time in days or weeks, you may be able to divert your attention from cigarettes to other pressing issues.

Factor in Your Addictive Profile

During Stage 2, the Entitlement Drive and the Defiance Drive are the most prominent, so you need to be vigilant if your scores for these drives showed an imbalance.

Entitlement Drive: As the weeks progress, you may find yourself living with a tempting and taunting option of smoking one puff to put an end to your struggle—especially if you've had a particularly hard day at the office or have been confronted with a stressful situation. The Entitlement Drive can wear away at your resolve like a spoiled child crying for a lollipop after a doctor's visit. Be ready with small rewards that don't involve tangible substances. For example, after a stressful day at work, treat yourself to a massage or a swim at the pool. Make a date to see a movie. Call a friend. Try to reconnect with activities that once gave you pleasure but which you've been avoiding because of your smoking habit.

Defiance Drive: If the Defiance Drive has been a factor in your habit, you may find it making a return visit as the weeks go by. In response to your discomfort, you may be tempted to say, "I don't have to put up with this misery. I'll do what I want." Instead, turn your defiance against your habit, making it work for you, not against you. Say, "I refuse to let this stick of tobacco run my life." You may be helped by joining a group where you can articulate your strong feelings in a supportive environment.

STAGE 3: FROM TWO TO THREE MONTHS

The transition between the second and the third stages is less dramatic than the one between the first and the second stages. The third stage lasts for two to three months. I have observed a rare, but strange, phenomenon where some smokers who appeared to be quite comfortable in the second stage found it harder to stay away from the habit when they entered the third stage. It is possible that these smokers had given up smoking for an explicit reason like recurrent bronchitis, which no longer existed a few weeks after the last puff. Once the reason disappears, the desire to smoke may return to haunt such individuals. But a majority of smokers experience a visible change in their outlook and establish a firm control over the habit.

There will be frequent, strong short bursts of memories about the cigarettes. Most of the time, these memories will be accompanied by a moderate desire to smoke, and occasionally a relatively strong desire to smoke which lasts for one to two minutes. An unexpected mishap like a flat tire or missing a train will trigger an urge to smoke, which may last for two to three minutes. You may express a slight desire to smoke, as you feel an emptiness in your chest. Even though you miss cigarettes, you can tolerate this level of discomfort.

The temptation to go back to smoking gradually subsides to a comfortable level toward the end of the third stage. Beware! Even though at the outset everything appears to be cool and calm, the volcano (smoking habit) can erupt at any time. A trivial, disappointing incident can immediately trigger a need to smoke. Most smokers escape without reaching for a cigarette, but such situations are a clear test of their resolve and commitment. Temptation to smoke a cigarette can also temporarily return under the influence of alcohol or mind-altering drugs.

Factor in Your Addictive Profile

During Stage 3, the Disenchantment Drive and the Invincibility Drive are the most prominent, so you need to be vigilant if your scores for these drives showed an imbalance.

Disenchantment Drive: Memories of the cigarettes are strong and constant. There will be a definite sense of loss of a good friend, followed by sadness. You may be touchy and sensitive. Rather than basking in your sadness, work to create a more pleasing environment. Focus on once again being able to appreciate a fine sense of smell and taste. Clean your house and car to rid them of any lingering traces of the smoking habit. A clean breath of fresh air, which most people take for granted, has been denied to you for a long time, but now it has been restored, and that can be a cause for great joy.

Invincibility Drive: The Invincibility Drive can be the hardest to conquer. The very fact that you have lasted several months without smoking can trigger a renewed sense of invincibility. You may feel that because you have succeeded, it's not so hard to quit whenever you want. You're in control. Don't allow these self-deceptive notions to creep in on you. Give yourself a reality check by watching a film or reading about the effects of smoking. Attend a lecture at your local hospital. Write in your journal about the benefits you've noticed of not smoking.

STAGE 4: FOUR MONTHS TO ONE YEAR

The fourth stage starts around the fourth month after the last puff, and without fanfare fades into the fifth and final stage by the end of one year. You may encounter an occasional twinge of desire to smoke, especially during occasions, such as the early morning, after dinner, or after sex, when you used to derive maximum pleasure from your habit. At times the memories of the habit, though not strong, will still distract your attention. But such memories usually are not accompanied by a desire to smoke. You will have a relatively easy time brushing off the urges.

At the end of this stage, you'll be almost free from the habit. By now, the pungent odor from cigarette ashes is as offensive to you as to all other nonsmokers. In fact, you may realize for the first time how difficult it must have been for other nonsmokers to bear the stench of your habit in the past. About 20 to 30 percent of ex-smokers may still go back to smoking after an interval of six to eight months. A nonsmoker wonders how a sensible person can fall into the same trap after struggling for months to get out of it! The answer is very simple: once an addictive habit has made an impression in the Emotional Division, it stays there forever. An addictive habit remains silent only against a conscious guard. Despite stern warnings from experts, smokers still flirt with the idea of smoking cigarettes and get into trouble.

Twelve months after the last puff, barring any unusual events, most smokers are ready to close the doors on cigarettes forever. These ex-smokers are looking forward to spending the rest of their lives in unprecedented, total freedom and tranquility.

STEP 5

Become a Comfortable Nonsmoker

YOUR GOAL IS to become a comfortable nonsmoker—that is, a person who no longer thinks about or desires a smoke. An uncomfortable nonsmoker is a person ready to return to the habit at the drop of a hat. Remember, comfort equals freedom. The following tips will help you achieve that wonderful state.

Avoid the Common Myths of Former Smokers

I train my patients to reject paying a heavy penalty in pursuit of a habit. They must choose to sacrifice the pleasure, thrill, or soothing effects derived from smoking. Initially, this seems like a tall order. After all, these are the very sticking points that have allowed the habit to have such power.

As you pursue a smoke-free life, be aware that there are land mines scattered over the terrain, invisible and waiting to explode. Let's examine the most dangerous.

Myth: You Can Return to the Lion's Den

It is foolish to think you can easily conquer your smoking habit if you continue the same patterns. Why put yourself in the way of such temptation? I am constantly amazed by people who tell me they can't understand why they failed to quit, then go on to say they continued to head for the same bar after work every day.

It will be enormously helpful if you simultaneously change the patterns of your day that aided and abetted your habit. Replace your sense of deprivation with positive action. For example, Helen, a fifty-eight-year-old office worker, wasn't able to smoke at work, so she really looked forward to her first after-work cigarette. It was the signal that she could relax and let her hair down.

Helen belonged to a gym, but like many people who make a commitment to exercise, she had let her membership lapse. I wanted Helen to rebuild a structured, disciplined routine and to break the physical cycle of her addiction. I instructed her to go directly from work to the gym, instead of going straight home. Exercising for an hour at the gym after work for five days a week would accomplish several things. First, it would help control her weight when she quit smoking. Second, boosting her endorphins through exercise would lift her mood, make her calmer, and raise her morale. She needed these changes to gain the strength to say no to cigarettes. It is a well-known fact that endorphins are a powerful natural antidepressant. Human manufactured chemical antidepressants are no match for the brain's natural endorphins when it comes to mood lifting.

I also advised Helen to drink lots of my favorite concoction—ice water with freshly squeezed lemon and a pinch of salt. There are a couple of reasons why I recommend this drink. Most smokers struggle with the absence of hand-to-mouth activity for at least a few days after they quit. Instead of eating rich foods or drinking high-calorie sodas and shakes, this beverage is pleasant and has an appealing taste compared with plain water. It has the added advantage of helping to flush the kidneys of toxins. (If you suffer from an ailment that restricts salt and water intake, check with your doctor before using this method.)

The physical break is a crucial first step, but it must be taken fully armed. A smoker who continues to hang out at his favorite bar, where he has always enjoyed a few cigarettes, is tempting the addiction's return—especially since alcohol will weaken his resolve. To break the habit, you must stop behaving habitually.

Myth: Replacement Substances Will Get You Through

Replacement substances of any kind, whether they are a nicotine patch or a toothpick in your mouth in place of a cigarette, are traps, because they keep your mind tuned into the habit. They are nothing more than expensive placebos that promote failure.

Sheryl, a thirty-nine-year-old patient, told me that the patch helped her stay away from cigarettes all day at work. But as soon as she went home, she had the urge to smoke. Her routine in the evening consisted of a nice hot bath, a sumptuous meal, and smoking six to eight cigarettes along with a couple of glasses of wine over a period of four hours. Sheryl found this evening ritual very gratifying, and cigarettes were an integral part of the routine. She didn't really care for the nicotine but definitely longed for the act of smoking in a special setting, and the patch could not fulfill the emotional need and the void created by the absence of this habit.

Two weeks after Sheryl's last puff, the withdrawal symptoms in the evening were severe and unbearable. As a desperate measure, she applied two 21-milligram nicotine patches in the evening, hoping that the increased nicotine level in her blood would eliminate the urges. To her dismay, this had no effect on her evening urges. After three weeks of fighting her strong desire to smoke, she finally caved in and went back to smoking. For a few months, Sheryl had an interesting relationship with the nicotine patch and cigarettes. During the day she would keep the patch on and stay away from cigarettes, but as soon as she got home, she would take off the patch and smoke to her heart's content. She felt that it was an excellent arrangement, but it did not last long, because the urge to smoke gradually crept up on her even during the daytime. In the end she gave up hope of quitting smoking through the nicotine-supplement technique.

After listening to Sheryl's story, I told her that until, and unless, she mentally agreed to forgo the pleasure she derived from the act of smoking, she would never overcome the urge and the withdrawal symptoms.

Myth: You Can Return to Being a Comfortable Occasional Smoker

Convincing yourself that one cigarette won't hurt you when you're on vacation or under great stress denies the reality that the habit is centered in the mind, not in the behavior. You cannot become a comfortable nonsmoker unless you reject the lie that smoking will bring comfort, pleasure, and satisfaction. Unfortunately, you cannot forget that there is a compelling, unyielding, powerful magnetic force generated by an addictive habit in the Emotional Division. The centrifugal force caused by the addictive habit will keep you going in circles forever, in a closed-loop orbit around its center.

Human behavior never ceases to amaze me. No matter how many times I tell my patients not to give in to the idea of bumming a smoke here and there after they've quit, many of them continue to toy with the idea of occasional consumption. Once they've been without cigarettes for a few weeks or months, they begin to second-guess the wisdom of giving up their favorite habit altogether. Maybe they start with one cigarette a day, or a couple of cigarettes a week. Sometimes they just take a puff or two and not even finish the cigarette. They grow confident that they are in control. But once the habit has a foothold, it only takes a bad day at the office or a fight with a partner to send the drive back to smoking in high gear.

Recently, I treated a forty-one-year-old female patient. Jeanine was thrilled when she successfully quit smoking, and she told me she felt no pressure to start again. Several months after she quit, she still assured me that she was a comfortable nonsmoker. I didn't hear from her after that until two years had passed. Jeanine arrived sheepishly in my office and confessed that she had gone back to smoking and wanted to try to quit again.

Naturally, I was curious about why she had gone back to smoking. "What drove you to pick up a cigarette after such a long absence?" I asked. Jeanine told me the following story.

One day she received a call at the office from the emergency room of a local hospital. She was informed that her eighteen-year-old son had been involved in a car accident. The person on the phone didn't give Jeanine any details, just told her to come to the ER as soon as possible. Naturally, Jeanine was stricken with fear for her son, and she raced to the hospital. On the way, her head filled with scenes of the worst-case scenarios. When she arrived at the hospital, she dashed into the emergency room. Immediately, before she even spoke to the nurse, Jeanine saw a man smoking in the lounge, and she bummed a cigarette off him. She was in a state of shock and did not realize what she was doing. Later, she repented her actions, but it was too late. The good news was that Jeanine's son had escaped the accident relatively unscathed. The bad news was that she went back to smoking. The anguish generated by this event demanded comfort and consolation, and this was met by her old friend, cigarettes. This is a slippery slope, my friends. There is no in between. Deep distress can instantly drive you to reach for the dormant addictive habit.

The mind is clever. It will contrive ways to return to the habit for which its affection and loyalty run deep. Even years after they've quit, I hear people express their displeasure toward the events or reasons that forced them to give up their favorite habit. They refuse to put their habit in the same league as alcohol or drugs. On some level, they maintain the myth of control. Ironically, the fact that they managed to quit smoking boosts their confidence in their ability to handle a smoke or two without sliding back. Inevitably, however, they slip into their old habit.

The ability to visualize negative consequences is an important factor in giving up a habit. Unfortunately, for a smoker the threat may be hidden. For example, there are many smokers who reach a ripe old age without experiencing any health problems. If an ex-smoker has not personally experienced a health problem, it is not easy for him to visualize the health risks associated with smoking. On the contrary, financial disasters, family disruptions, or a threat to employment, as well as the legal hassles imposed by alcohol and hard-drug usage, are certainly much easier to visualize and to remember for a onetime alcoholic or drug addict.

Out of curiosity, I conducted an unofficial follow-up study to determine the number of people from various addiction groups who had given up their respective habits but had gone back to them a year later. These were not my own patients, but blindly selected volunteers. The study group included smokers, alcoholics, and hard-drug (cocaine, heroin) users. All of the participants came from upper- and middle-class families. They all gave up the addiction on their own with considerable hardship. One year later, 56 percent of the smokers, 45 percent of the alcoholics, and 35 percent of the hard-drug addicts had gone back to their addictions. The results were quite surprising, to say the least. One would have expected a much higher percentage of hard-drug addicts to return to their habits compared to smokers and alcoholics, because cocaine and heroin generate a stronger chemical hold and a more compelling desire than nicotine or alcohol. But this was not the case. Cigarettes won out every time.

The bottom line: respect the power of this addiction and don't kid yourself that you can be an occasional smoker.

Meditation: Summoning the Mind's Healing Energy

Keeping your mind strong and supple will help you maintain your nonsmoker status and reduce your stress during the battle to quit. Meditation can help you summon your mind's healing energy, and retrieve your mind from a war zone and place it in a neutral zone.

The objective of meditation is more important than the steps you take to get there. Meditating is not about disconnecting from the world around you. It is not about shutting off your five senses and making your mind passive in order to reduce stress. It won't work. Stress is the most annoying, adept, persistent pest— like a cockroach of the mind. Cockroaches, as we know, have an extraordinary ability to survive by defying all attempts to eradicate them. Stress is in the same league. It will not cave in to such feeble tactics. For this you need big guns. However, stress can be somewhat alleviated if you grasp and practice the true concept of meditation.

Meditation involves stepping back from this world for a short period. While you turn off your five senses, you must turn on the internal sense that connects you with nature through your instincts. Meditation is not a passive state of mind. On the contrary, your mind will be in its most active state—more authentically than ever. Connecting with nature involves understanding its mandates about life and accepting its truth about your place in the world. This is both an exhilarating and humbling experience.

Every time I meditate, I pick one or two issues in my life and strive to understand the full truth about them—not only how I perceive them but also nature's truth about them. Only then can I resolve the issues. This practice is relevant to the smoker. Not only must you consider your perspective, you must also strive to discover nature's truth—that if you continue to smoke, you will suffer consequences. Accepting nature's truth will help you rise above the discomfort involved in quitting and embrace your full potential.

Meditation is a tool that can alleviate stress and strengthen your sense of purpose and will. But the process is not magical. You have to be open to seeing life as it really is, not as you want it to be. You have to choose priorities that elevate you, as opposed to the deceitful and destructive priorities you once held.

EXERCISE: VISUALIZE YOURSELF AT PEACE AND IN CONTROL

Sit in a comfortable position. Allow your arms to rest at your sides, palms of hands up. Inhale and exhale slowly and deeply, keeping your eyes closed. Focus on the rhythm of your breathing and the movement of your abdomen and lungs as the healing energy flows through you. As you exhale, say the word "peace" to yourself, drawing it out as one long breath: p-e-e-a-a-a-c-c-c-e-e-e. Visualize your anxiety like a bird, and watch it fly away as you breathe in and out and repeat the peace mantra. Continue for at least five minutes or until you feel relaxed.

FREQUENCY AND DURATION

In the beginning, meditating once a day is enough. However, over the years the strong, positive mental high will become natural. Eventually, even a brief meditation each day will keep you in good spirits throughout the day and allow you to face what comes your way as a challenge, not as a chore.

Time of Day

Find a time when you can comfortably spare thirty minutes or so without interruption. It can be any time of day. For me, early morning is best. I like to pool my energy and strength before I leap into the day's tasks.

Location

Find a place without distraction—a quiet room in your home, a nearby park, or even a parking space in an empty shopping mall

WHEN ARE ANTI-ANXIETY MEDICATIONS NECESSARY?

I strongly urge my patients to strive to relax naturally through meditation. Realistically, however, I understand that a small percentage of extremely entrenched smokers may need short-term extra help from anti-anxiety medications such as Elavil, Xanax, or Buspirone. If you find that your anxiety levels are getting the best of you, talk to your doctor about a prescription—but I encourage you to use the medication for only seven days.

lot. Don't carry your cell phone or beeper. A small Walkman or MP3 player with appealing music is fine.

Maintain a Healthy Weight

Many people gain weight after giving up smoking, and there is a great deal of misunderstanding about why that occurs. Most people believe that nicotine accelerates the metabolism and helps them control their weight. I can confidently say that this belief is not true. After all, nicotine is a mild stimulant. In its absence, the resultant metabolic changes—which are minimal and momentary—may account for 1 to 2 percent of weight gain.

Any weight gain over this percentage is not caused by increased appetite but is due to a substitution factor. In the beginning, there is a great need to keep the mouth and hands busy. Naturally, food comes in very handy as a safe substitute. In reality, food or any other substitute does not fill the void left by the absence of cigarettes, so the smoker continues to eat, instead of picking up a cigarette. Another reason ex-smokers may begin to eat more is that after giving up smoking, the improved appreciation of smell and taste for food increases their appetite and as a result the amount of food they consume. These altered eating routines are responsible for the weight gain. A successful nonsmoker can avoid the weight gain by eschewing the metabolic factor and implementing measures such as daily exercise and eating balanced meals.

If you gain a lot of weight within three to four weeks after the last puff, it is due to a direct substitution for cigarettes. However, if the weight gain is more gradual, it's likely that you're just tasting the food more fully than before. Improved taste and smell reception may produce a greater desire to eat. It's that simple.

Many of my patients, especially women, are panicked when they experience weight gain, and they're tempted to go back to smoking. I remind them that the weight they gained after they quit smoking will stick with them even if they return to smoking, since only a tiny percentage is associated with metabolic changes. Furthermore, studies show that individuals using the nicotine patch tend to eat more than usual.

Weight gain is a prelude to failure. It indicates that you have given up cigarettes, but not the smoking habit. You're looking for comfort from sources other than cigarettes. If you're replacing cigarettes with food, because the craving for some kind of crutch still exists, you need to evaluate that in the context of your addictive drives.

When you follow my method, and break your habit from the inside out, you will be less likely to overeat as a compensation. In the process of addressing your addictive drives, you will feel a new power over all of your compulsions. You will realize that you *can* help yourself. You are no longer a victim to the urge to smoke—or to overeat.

STEP 6

Eliminate the Mentality
of Addiction

ADDICTION IS a form of slavery, and the goal should be freedom. Unfortunately, the current culture of "recovery" promotes the idea of "once a smoker, always a smoker." Many of my patients tell me that their greatest desire is to be completely free of smoking—to feel no tug of desire toward their old habit whatsoever. Is this possible?

This is where I part ways with the Twelve Step ideology, which many smoking-cessation programs are now using. The Twelve Step method encourages smokers to think of their addictions as permanent—like dormant bombs set to explode without warning. Constant vigilance is required. What a drag! In my experience, what addicts really long for is normalcy—the state of comfortable non-addiction—not continued obsession. After all, their addiction has already stolen years from their lives. When they look at themselves in the mirror, they don't want to say, "I am a smoker in recovery." Such a pronouncement can do little more than sap the spirit. Likewise, to say, "I am a former smoker" has a very different effect on one's psychology than to say, "I am a nonsmoker." I've noticed that most people who've kicked the smoking habit cannot answer the question, "Do you smoke?" with a simple, unambiguous "No."

Recently I listened to a radio program describing the success of a New Jersey hospital program that helped people stop smoking, using a combination of group therapy and antidepressants. The program boasted a remarkable success rate; after three months, the majority of the participants had completely kicked their smoking habits. Several of the participants were interviewed on the radio program, and I particularly remember one woman, who proudly announced herself to be smoke-free before adding, "But I would kill for a cigarette."

Through the emotional adjustment, most people are able to control the desire to seek comfort from habits on a day-to-day basis. However, they almost always say they carry a deep dread of what will occur the first time they experience a highly stressful situation. They don't trust their instincts to choose a different, more productive method of relief—probably because they've "fallen off the wagon" so many times in the past.

If you are to be successful in conquering your enemy, you must face your habit without fear. That is possible with the inside-out approach. It is not possible with the outside-in approach.

Eliminating the mentality of addiction is the most crucial step in the process—the one that makes change permanent. How is it accomplished? Remember, the Instinctual Division of the mind is not independent of the Intellectual and Emotional divisions. The instinct to reach for a cigarette in times of stress is a learned behavior. Even when the Emotional Division is no longer demanding the relief, the Instinctual Division must be reconfigured to respond differently. In essence, it must be trained to have an alternative automatic response to stress.

We all face obstacles in life regularly. Sometimes we are distressed, upset, disappointed, or hurt. Being treated unfairly by others hurts us the most. Believe it or not, it happens to us all the time. Pain and anguish demand immediate compensation. We need to do something to soothe the pain at that moment of distress. We take an inventory of what activities have given or could give us relief and comfort on such occasions. Usually, addictive habits are at the top of that list, and we go for them, even if we have once parted with them. Your task will be to evaluate the other items on that list, which you can use instead.

My patients who use the inside-out approach to quitting are amazed by how little they are bothered in the presence of cigarettes. As one of them told me, "A week after I quit, my friend who smokes hesitated to light up in front of me. I told her to go ahead, that I didn't care. To my surprise her smoking reminded me that I once smoked and used to enjoy it, but now I don't care for it anymore."

Feeling so free of the power of cigarettes is a tremendous relief to people. Once you make the mental break, you are not afraid that you'll slip. My patients tell me that they get rid of the ashtrays and other smoking paraphernalia in their homes, not because they're afraid of slipping but because they find the stench offensive.

Close the Door—Forever

I ask my patients to perform visualization exercises—to picture themselves at the final moment when they close the door on their smoking habit and lock it behind them. Some have difficulty looking ahead; others balk at locking the door. Still others experience a sudden urge to take one last look. This exercise is immensely powerful. It completes the emotional adjustment. Closing the door, placing a sturdy lock on it, and throwing away the key, the individual bids a lasting farewell to the habit, with no possibility of returning. If all of the previous steps have been completed, the process feels completely natural.

As you begin to see yourself and your place in the world in a more realistic light, these priorities will emerge naturally: peace of mind, unadulterated good health, freedom, and the natural high that comes from being at one with nature. When your priorities are straight, everything else falls into place. You may still strive to make good money, but the desire for money won't run you. You may seek material comforts, but not need them for your well-being. Your relationships will occur naturally on your own terms; you will no longer feel the need to create facades to make yourself more popular.

At first this may seem to be totally beside the point of whether you smoke or not. But it is intimately related. The drive to smoke is a manifestation of slavery, and there are many kinds of slavery.

When I was an adolescent, my mother, a very wise woman, told me, "Don't ever chase after fame or fortune. You will become their slave."

I was a sassy young man, so I replied, "You have told me what *not* to do, but you haven't told me what *to* do."

She smiled at me and replied, "Simple. Keep your priorities straight and strong. Never try to compete with your fellow human beings, only with yourself. Bring the best you have to offer to every day, and let nature take its course. I promise you, if you do this, fame and fortune will chase after you, but they will never own you. Instead you will own them."

My mother's advice stayed with me. I wanted this freedom. That is one reason I do the work I do—to show others the way out of their slavery.

Be a Happy Nonsmoker—for Good

A patient walks into my office for help quitting smoking, usually after many failed attempts. Yet I do not talk to this person about cigarettes, or discuss how many packs a day are being smoked, or lecture about the damage to my patient's health. Instead, I say, "You have an enemy who is bent on destroying you, and you feel helpless to do anything about it. You can reverse the tide, stop the enemy dead in its tracks, and beat it to a pulp by no longer feeling helpless." What I have to offer is a winning strategy, not a losing proposition.

My patients usually look at me hopefully, as if thinking I have a magic formula that will get them out of the mess they're in. I tell them, "I am a physician, not a magician." I don't blame people for seeking the easiest way out of their dilemma. Who wouldn't want to conquer a great enemy with the snap of the fingers? But it just doesn't work that way. Our Maker has sent us out to a battleground, not a playground. If you want to quit smoking, you have to confront the enemy on its own turf. There is no other way. I don't make the rules. Nature does.

We come to the world alone. We fight our battles alone. We endure the consequences alone. We die alone. This is the way it is for every human being. So the first order of business is to fully know this self. This may seem like an automatic task, but that is not the case. Usually, our vision is so clouded with the collective opinions of the world that we allow ourselves to be defined by the judgments of others. Self-evaluation involves stripping off the layers of cover-up and analyzing our prospects with an unfaltering eye.

My patients, especially those trying to overcome addictions, often ask me, "Where will I find the strength to live on my own?" There is only one answer to that question. You must all find strength within. No external source can give you strength. Once you internalize that understanding, there is nothing to stop you.

Ultimate satisfaction is the knowledge that you have lived a successful life. What is a successful life, and how can you be assured of leading one? In my opinion, a successful individual is able to leave this world with a broad, contented smile, knowing that he has led a productive, stress-free life by utilizing his talents and opportunities to the fullest extent.

APPENDIX
Frequently Asked Questions

Is it really possible to quit by following the method in this book? Don't people need hands-on treatment or support?

Obviously reading a book is a bit different than seeking personal treatment. For those who are strongly motivated to quit, and don't have large barriers, the book will be enough. Others may need more help. But I strongly believe that using the book to take your solitary journey is a good start. Remember, you alone can overcome your habit. Not a support group or a therapist. Just you.

Do you offer more than your philosophy and strategies to your patients?

Yes, I do. I guide my patients through two steps. First, all patients are exposed to the concepts I have outlined in this book. Many times that is sufficient for an individual to part with his habit. To complete this step, a patient will visit me from one to three times, depending on the number of drives that control his habit. Second, my patients receive special hands-on treatments, which I have devised to offer a head start for true, hard-core addicts who have lost confidence in their ability to quit. Usually this step takes two or three treatments over a period of ten to fifteen days. These treatments boost the patient's confidence, conviction, and level of tolerance to emotional discomfort, thereby allowing him to conquer his archenemy—the smoking habit.

What about snuff or chewing tobacco? Are they as harmful as cigarettes?

Snuff is flavored, fine tobacco powder. The usual method is to periodically sniff a pinch of the tobacco. Depending upon the size of the pinch, between 1 and 2 milligrams is delivered into the nasal mucous membrane, from which it is rapidly absorbed into the bloodstream. In addition to feeling a slight stimulation, snuff users also experience a ticklish sensation in the nose, followed by a bout of sneezing. Many have told me that the attractive ticklish sensation followed by dizzy spells entices them to this habit.

Sniffing snuff is not nearly as common as smoking cigarettes, but the dangers can be just as great. Long-term usage of snuff leads to drying of the nasal passages, frequent nosebleeds, polyps, and ultimately cancer of the nasal passages.

Chewing tobacco is an age-old tradition in many Eastern countries. In India, people are in the habit of chewing a mixture of coarsely shredded tobacco with a pinch of limestone powder (calcium hydroxide) for extra kicks. Apparently, nicotine is released faster if it is chewed in this fashion. Most addicts use a wad of shredded tobacco tucked in their cheek, but some use a different method called dipping, where a pinch of snuff is placed between the lower lip and the gum. Depending upon the size of the wad or the pinch, up to 6 milligrams of nicotine is delivered within thirty minutes. Many tobacco chewers are ill informed about the risks of their habit. Among the dangers are gingivitis, leading to premature loss of teeth; stomach inflammation, which leads to ulcers and cancer; and oral cancer.

Do men or women have a harder time quitting?

In my experience, there are minimal differences in the performance and the success ratio between men and women. There are a few exceptions to this rule. Loneliness affects women more often than men. For example, a fifty-five-year-old single male, either a widower or a divorcé, will tend to tolerate the ordeal of giving up smoking far better than a female. If a couple attempts to give up smoking at the same time, the female's chances of staying off the cigarettes hinges more on her male counterpart. But the reverse is not true. Men have a higher threshold to withstand personal tragedies compared to women but lose their cool easily to business and professional upheavals. On the other hand, women falter on personal issues and relationship problems. I've also noticed that women seem to miss cigarettes more than men and are more likely to go through a spell of sadness or depression immediately after the last puff. Men are more likely to be irritable than women for the first few days after giving up smoking.

You mentioned earlier that you are not a total fan of the Twelve Step ideology. Why is this true?

No doubt Twelve Step programs have helped many addicts. I do concur with a few of the Twelve Step premises but disagree with them on many more. For example, the Twelve Step ideology agrees that addiction is a problem of the mind, not the brain. We both believe in correcting the behavior of an addict through outlook and attitude rather than tweaking the brain chemistry. Where we disagree is on the methods needed for recovery. For instance:

- The Twelve Step ideology states that it takes a collective effort to control addiction. I believe in individual effort. I'm not saying one can't have support from family and friends. But the key for all addicts rests in their own mind and will.

- The Twelve Step ideology treats the addict as a powerless weakling who cannot handle the addiction alone. I believe this is a cheap excuse. If an individual is not willing to fight back against his addiction and take control of his life, he is a lost cause. No amount of support, sympathy, empathy, and hand-holding will make a lasting difference. From the outset I encourage the individual to see the facts clearly, to acknowledge personal responsibility, and to act independently of others.

- The Twelve Step ideology encourages a constant, long-term relationship with the addiction. It becomes an indispensable crutch, thereby fostering dependence, weakness, and insecurity. For the addict it is a choice between bonding to the group or being in control of the addiction. Maybe the group seems like the lesser of two evils, but neither is good for the spirit of an individual. I make sure my patients understand that our relationship is temporary, and the sooner they break away, the better.

- The Twelve Step ideology tries to ease the struggle by shielding the individual addict from the blows and bruises of his addiction. For example, if a person falls off the wagon, the Twelve Step program responds with sympathy for how tough the challenge is and forgives the person who slipped. Further, the individual is encouraged to forgive himself and pick up the pieces to start all over again. Unfortunately, nature is not so forgiving. The reality is that the first attempt to overcome an addiction is the easiest. Every subsequent attempt gets harder. Practice in the fight against addiction only makes the fight tougher. That is the reason I tell my patients, "Don't *try* to stop smoking. Do it! You may not get a second chance."

- The Twelve Step ideology contends that conquering addiction is a lifelong struggle. An addict is expected to set aside a good deal of time and energy fighting the battle for the rest of his life. But a lifelong struggle of any kind is debilitating. It dampens one's spirits. I encourage my patients to bring closure to their struggle and move forward, attending to their essential needs and possibilities. I tell them to look back only to appreciate how far they've come and to feel proud of their achievements. It is good for the soul and the spirit to close that chapter forever.

- Finally, the Twelve Step ideology is based on the premise that the addict is powerless over his addictions. In truth, an addict is not powerless over addiction, and he never was. He intentionally invited this scourge because at the time it was pleasurable, soothing, or thrilling. It helped him escape from a harsh reality. It is the addict's careless, immature, and irresponsible nature that has made his life unmanageable. If we say he is powerless, there is no way he can fight a winning battle. I hold my patients accountable for their addictions and related problems. I tell them that they are the perpetrators, not the victims, of their circumstances. This is a crucial first step toward recovery. I agree that there is a power in the universe that is greater than all of us. However, I do not believe our Maker will restore us to sanity, if we only place ourselves passively in His hands. Believing in our Maker means accepting the terms and conditions of nature and taking charge of our own actions.

Do people who are down on their luck or struggling financially have a harder time breaking bad habits?

Not necessarily. The key is what's going on inside. My patients are often men and women of great privilege. They are wealthy, successful, the envy of their peers. They have it all. They are also people who are trapped by addictions—to smoking, alcohol, food, drugs, gambling, sex—or haunted by debilitating fears and phobias. In them I observe the paradox of human behavior. On the one hand, my patients are smart and powerful. On the other hand, they are foolish and destructive. They have won the lottery of life, yet they are disappointed. They have failed to take full measure of themselves—who they are and what is possible for them. Instead, most of them define themselves by the way the world treats them. This is the source of much suffering and wasted energy. They worry about deficiencies that only exist in the eyes of the world.

What about aids to help stop smoking?

Addictive behaviors cannot be overcome by tweaking chemicals in the brain, although such approaches are very seductive because they take the responsibility for the addiction away from the individual and place it on chemistry. The addiction is thus objectified in the same way that a blood disease or a thyroid disorder might be objectified. The cure is presented as a simple matter of rewiring the brain—or of altering the chemical environment of the brain. But if it were that simple, why would so many people fail to rid themselves of their destructive habits?

Here is the truth of the matter, which I have learned from treating thousands of patients. Almost every individual is able to stop smoking for a short time. The people who come to me have all done this. Smokers have put down cigarettes for a week or two; some have even quit for a year or more before returning to the habit. If it were a matter of chemistry alone, that would be the end of it. But usually smokers tell me that during these periods of abstinence, their minds are consumed with the desire for a cigarette. They do not think of themselves as nonsmokers; the habit lingers in their minds.

My method is based on the understanding that addictive behavior is driven by an imbalance in the divisions of the mind, not the chemicals in the brain.

What do you think is the greatest barrier to people giving up bad habits?

Arrogance is the greatest barrier to fulfillment. It will stop you dead in your tracks. You are not God. You are not omnipotent. There is great power in acknowledging your place in the world, but many people cannot see this because they are obsessed with what others think. Recently I was treating a young man who had a heroin addiction. Before he became addicted, he was quite successful, earning a very high salary. Now he was not working, and his mother was paying for his treatment. I asked him, "Why are you allowing your mother to pay your way?" He replied, "The only jobs I can get these days are too demeaning. I'm accustomed to making a salary in the six figures, and I refuse to settle for a menial job. I have my pride."

I told this young man, "Your pride is killing you. You are faced with a most important matter of your survival on this planet, and you refuse to accept reality. You cannot have the job you had before. It is not being offered to you. There are only two options. You can view the job being offered as demeaning, which will prevent you from succeeding, or you can determine to make the most of it and see where it takes you."

Is it better to be public about the decision to quit smoking or to keep it private?

Some smokers may elect to face this challenge on their own in seclusion. If a smoker decides to keep the attempt a secret, he doesn't have to worry about facing public humiliation if he falters. Some smokers also report they are able to focus better on their efforts when the world is not watching.

Others do well in a public forum, believing that an open declaration of their intention compels them to work harder and win this game to save face. They should be cautious, as the strategy may backfire. Instead of strengthening a smoker's resolve, the anticipation of a humiliating defeat in front of friends and relatives may intensify pressure on the smoker, raising anxiety levels and undermining success. Even a well-meaning inquiry of their progress from friends and family members may be construed as an offensive intrusion. The preoccupation of an impending ridicule and shame may prevent a smoker from focusing on the objectives of the task ahead. Finally, the enthusiasm to succeed may be replaced by the fear of failure and anguish. A smoker's ability to hit the smoking habit hard is automatically diminished if he fails to relax and compose his thoughts properly, just before the final confrontation.

It is an excellent idea if a group of smokers chooses to stop smoking together with the intention of helping one another. If the individual members of the group handle the situation delicately, they have more to gain from this strategy than attempting it on their own.

How can I make sure that my children do not pick up the smoking habit?

My mother often said, "There are many intelligent people in this world, but there are few smart people." Kids today must be smart to avoid the pressure to use drugs, smoke, or drink alcohol. As parents, you can play a crucial role in helping them to be smarter.

First, know that actions speak louder than words. If you smoke, your moral authority is zero. Many parents complain that their kids don't pay any attention to what they do or say. This is absolutely wrong. You are a more important influence on your children than their peers or all the forces of society they encounter outside the home.

Second, take an inside-out approach. You can lecture them about smoking until kingdom come, but it will have little effect if the inner building blocks are not there. Help your children to develop strong self-esteem and inner resolve so they won't become ruled by the addictive profiles. Teach them that happiness and a sense of purpose come from within; they are not given to them by others or achieved through crutches like smoking. Enable them to understand the blunt realities of nature—that if they make mistakes, nature issues consequences. Show them through your words and actions that a fulfilling, exuberant life can be achieved. When they see you living with joy, they will want to emulate you.

You are so passionate about your work. Where did you learn your philosophy? Did it evolve from your own experiences?

I am an ordinary human being, just like everyone else, and I wasn't always such a happy camper. I found my vision through my struggles. Let me tell you the experience that changed my life.

I was born in India, a country of deprivation, and yet I grew up in comfort. All my life I was treated like a prince. And so, when I left India to pursue a medical residency in England, I was full of arrogance. My attitude was, "I am doing you a great favor by coming here. You need me more than I need you. I am special."

When I arrived in England, with my young wife in tow, I expected the red carpet treatment. I applied to the top programs, both in neurosurgery and in cardiothoracic surgery—and one after the other, I was rejected. I was accepted into only one program, which was not the one I wanted. It was a psychiatry residency.

I was angry. I felt disillusioned, betrayed, lost. My first reaction was, "You can't treat me this way. I'm going home." But one night, hours before I was scheduled to leave, I had a realization. For the first time in my life I was confronted with a challenge, and what was my response? To run back to safety.

I took a hard look at myself. "Balasa, you think you are better than everyone else. You think you have something special to offer. You are not special. No one is special. Nature does not treat you like a special case. You need this world as much as this world needs you. Don't you forget that."

That night I decided I would not run away. I would stay and fight.

I signed up for the psychiatric residency. My humiliation woke me up. I crashed into the absolute truth of Almighty Nature. Not the way I wished it would be. The way it was. Almighty Nature—or God, or whatever you call the great force of the universe—has its rules. It's up to us to figure them out. There are no free rides. No special circumstances. So I took what was available to me. But then I saw I had another choice to make. I could embrace the challenge fully, or I could be halfhearted, bitching all the way. I chose. I said, "I am going to put my heart and soul into this psychiatric residency." And that is when I crossed the line between merely accepting my fate and using my fate to create my masterpiece.

My work became exhilarating and fulfilling. It was not the ending point. It was the beginning point. In the coming years, I was able to build on my clinical training to give me insight into the mind and body from different perspectives. After completing a residency in psychiatry, I pursued residencies in internal medicine and family medicine to better grasp the association between body, mind, and behavior. When I moved to the United States in 1972, I took on a fourth residency in anesthesia, to study the influence of powerful analgesics, hypnotics, and tranquilizers. By the time I opened my practice in behavior modification, I had developed a system that integrated the Eastern wisdom of my heritage with the vast potential of Western technology.

I persevered in my profession because I had learned the lesson of humility: *Ask not what the world can do for you. Ask what you can do for yourself.* Life presents an opportunity. Find out what you can do with it. I have found a way to be master of my destiny. I have found peace of mind, clarity of mission. My message to you is simple: if I can do it, so can you.

INDEX